T0290648

PAIN MEDICINE
A CASE-BASED
LEARNING SERIES

Headache and Facial Pain

PAIN MEDICINE
A CASE-BASED LEARNING SERIES

Headache and Facial Pain

STEVEN D. WALDMAN, MD, JD

ELSEVIER

Elsevier
1600 John F. Kennedy Blvd.
Ste 1800
Philadelphia, PA 19103-2899

PAIN MEDICINE: A CASE-BASED LEARNING SERIES   ISBN: 978-0-323-83456-8
HEADACHE AND FACIAL PAIN

Notice

Practitioners and researchers must always rely on their own experience and knowledge in evaluating and using any information, methods, compounds or experiments described herein. Because of rapid advances in the medical sciences, in particular, independent verification of diagnoses and drug dosages should be made. To the fullest extent of the law, no responsibility is assumed by Elsevier, authors, editors or contributors for any injury and/or damage to persons or property as a matter of products liability, negligence or otherwise, or from any use or operation of any methods, products, instructions, or ideas contained in the material herein.

Executive Content Strategist: Michael Houston
Content Development Specialist: Jeannine Carrado/Laura Klein
Director, Content Development: Ellen Wurm-Cutter
Publishing Services Manager: Shereen Jameel
Senior Project Manager: Karthikeyan Murthy
Design Direction: Amy Buxton

Printed in India.

Last digit is the print number: 9 8 7 6 5 4 3 2 1

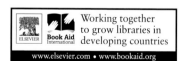

Working together to grow libraries in developing countries

www.elsevier.com • www.bookaid.org

To Peanut and David H.

SDW

"When you go after honey with a balloon, the great thing is to not let the bees know you're coming."

WINNIE THE POOH

It's Harder Than It Looks
MAKING THE CASE FOR CASE-BASED LEARNING

For sake of full disclosure, I was one of those guys. You know, the ones who wax poetic about how hard it is to teach our students how to do procedures. Let me tell you, teaching folks how to do epidurals on women in labor certainly takes its toll on the coronary arteries. It's true, I am amazing. . .I am great. . .I have nerves of steel. Yes, I could go on like this for hours. . .but you have heard it all before. But, it's again that time of year when our new students sit eagerly before us, full of hope and dreams. . .and that harsh reality comes slamming home. . .it is a lot harder to teach beginning medical students "doctoring" than it looks.

A few years ago, I was asked to teach first-year medical and physician assistant students how to take a history and perform a basic physical exam. In my mind, I thought, "This should be easy. . .no big deal," I won't have to do much more than show up. After all, I was the guy who wrote that amazing book on physical diagnosis. After all, I had been teaching medical students, residents, and fellows how to do highly technical (and dangerous, I might add) interventional pain management procedures since right after the Civil War. Seriously, it was no big deal. . .I could do it in my sleep. . .with one arm tied behind my back. . .blah. . .blah. . .blah.

For those of you who have had the privilege of teaching "doctoring," you already know what I am going to say next. *It's harder than it looks!* Let me repeat this to disabuse any of you who, like me, didn't get it the first time. *It is harder than it looks!* I only had to meet with my first-year medical and physician assistant students a couple of times to get it through my thick skull: **It really is harder than it looks**. In case you are wondering, the reason that our students look back at us with those blank, confused, bored, and ultimately dismissive looks is simple: They lack context. That's right, they lack the context to understand what we are talking about.

It's really that simple. . .or hard. . .depending on your point of view or stubbornness, as the case may be. To understand why context is king, you have to look only as far as something as basic as the Review of Systems. The Review of Systems is about as basic as it gets, yet why is it so perplexing to our students? Context. I guess it should come as no surprise to anyone that the student is completely lost when you talk about. . .let's say. . .the "constitutional" portion of the Review of Systems, without the context of what a specific constitutional finding, say a fever or chills, might mean to a patient who is suffering from the acute onset of headaches. If you tell the student that you need to ask about fever, chills, and the other "constitutional" stuff and you take it no further, you might as well be talking about the

International Space Station. Just save your breath; it makes absolutely no sense to your students. Yes, they want to please, so they will memorize the elements of the Review of Systems, but that is about as far as it goes. On the other hand, if you presented the case of Jannette Patton, a 28-year-old first-year medical resident with a fever and headache, you can see the lights start to come on. By the way, this is what Jannette looks like, and as you can see, Jannette is sicker than a dog. This, at its most basic level, is what *Case-Based Learning* is all about.

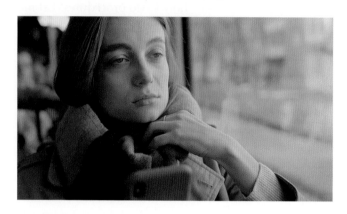

I would like to tell you that, smart guy that I am, I immediately saw the light and became a convert to *Case-Based Learning*. But truth be told, it was COVID-19 that really got me thinking about *Case-Based Learning*. Before the COVID-19 pandemic, I could just drag the students down to the med/surg wards and walk into a patient room and riff. Everyone was a winner. For the most part, the patients loved to play along and thought it was cool. The patient and the bedside was all I needed to provide the context that was necessary to illustrate what I was trying to teach—the "why headache and fever don't mix" kind of stuff. Had COVID-19 not rudely disrupted my ability to teach at the bedside, I suspect that you would not be reading this *Preface*, as I would not have had to write it. Within a very few days after the COVID-19 pandemic hit, my days of bedside teaching disappeared, but my students still needed context. This got me focused on how to provide the context they needed. The answer was, of course, *Case-Based Learning*. What started as a desire to provide context. . .because it really was **harder than it looked**. . .led me to begin work on this eight-volume *Case-Based Learning* textbook series. What you will find within these volumes are a bunch of fun, real-life cases that help make each patient come alive for the student. These cases provide the contextual teaching points that make it easy for the teacher to explain why, when Jannette's chief complaint is, *"My head is killing me and I've got a fever,"* it is a big deal.

Have fun!

Steven D. Waldman, MD, JD
Spring 2021

ACKNOWLEDGEMENTS

A very special thanks to my editors, Michael Houston, PhD, Jeannine Carrado, and Karthikeyan Murthy, for all of their hard work and perseverance in the face of disaster. Great editors such as Michael, Jeannine, and Karthikeyan make their authors look great, for they not only understand how to bring the Three Cs of great writing. . .Clarity + Consistency + Conciseness. . .to the author's work, but unlike me, they can actually punctuate and spell!

Steven D. Waldman, MD, JD

P.S. . . .Sorry for all the ellipses, guys!

ACKNOWLEDGMENTS

CONTENTS

Renaldo Saldana

A 58-Year-Old Male With Left-Sided Facial Pain and Rash

LEARNING OBJECTIVES

- Learn the common causes of facial pain.
- Learn the common types of painful rashes.
- Develop an understanding of varicella zoster infection.
- Learn the clinical presentation of shingles.
- Develop an understanding of the treatment options for shingles.
- Learn the appropriate testing options to help diagnose shingles.
- Learn to identify red flags in patients who present with acute facial pain.
- Develop an understanding of postherpetic neuralgia.

Renaldo Saldana

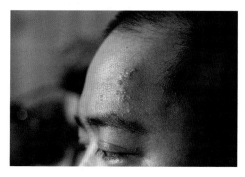

Renaldo Saldana is a 58 y/o waiter with the chief complaint of, "My left forehead is killing me." Renaldo went on to say that he wouldn't have bothered coming in just for the pain, which had been present for a couple of days, but when he developed a rash on his left forehead, his boss told him he couldn't wait tables and would have to wash dishes until the rash went away. I asked Renaldo if he had anything like this happen before. He shook his head and responded, "You know me, Doc, I am happy and healthy, but I am really worried about this rash. The damn forehead pain was bad enough, but when I woke up and saw this rash, it really freaked me out!" He continued, "Doc, the crazy thing is that the rash wasn't there when I went to bed. I am positive about this because I went to look in the bathroom mirror to see if I could see why my forehead was hurting, and there was nothing there. I get up this morning, and I see a couple of little blisters over my eye. Now the damn rash is spreading and my boss won't let me work. I'm pretty tough, but this really has me worried because if I don't work, I don't eat. The other crazy thing is it hurts when I try to comb my hair. What is that all about? Do you think I got bit by one of those brown recluse spiders?"

I asked Renaldo about any antecedent trauma to the forehead and he just shook his head. "Doc, this kind of snuck up on me. Like I said, at first, my forehead began aching and then I woke up with this crazy rash. But, like I also said, I gotta work." I asked Renaldo what made his pain worse and he said, "Anytime I forget and touch my forehead, it really hurts." He added, "You know, Doc, the other crazy thing is that if the fan in my room blows on my forehead, I get these sharp pains. What the hell is that about?"

I asked Renaldo to point with one finger to show me where it hurts the most. He pointed to the rash over his left eye, taking care not to touch the area. "Doc, I can't really point to one place. It kind of hurts all around my left eye and my forehead, and another crazy thing is, sometimes I feel like my hair hurts." I asked if he had any fever or chills and he shook his head no. I then asked, "What about steroids? Did you ever take any cortisone or drugs like that?" Renaldo again shook his head no. He denied any cancer or human immunodeficiency virus (HIV). Renaldo said, "Doc, you know me, I am happy and healthy," but with a worried look, he added, "This really has me freaked out. I really need your help!"

On physical examination, Renaldo was afebrile. His respirations were 18 and his pulse was 84 and regular. His blood pressure (BP) was slightly elevated at 144/88. I made a note to recheck it again before he left because he was pretty anxious. He had obvious vesicular lesions over the left eye. He had no lesions in his ear and both his eyes looked normal. His cardiopulmonary examination was unremarkable other than the mild hypertension. His thyroid was normal. His abdominal examination revealed no abnormal mass or organomegaly. There was no costovertebral angle (CVA) tenderness. There was no peripheral edema or adenopathy. His low back examination was unremarkable. I did a rectal exam, which revealed no mass and a normal prostate. The remainder of Renaldo's physical examination was within normal limits.

Key Clinical Points—What's Important and What's Not

THE HISTORY

- A history of left forehead pain, which occurred prior to the onset of vesicular rash
- No history of acute trauma
- No history of previous significant facial pain
- No fever or chills
- Acute onset of vesicular pain in the distribution of the left ophthalmic branch of the trigeminal nerve (V1) following the onset of forehead pain
- Allodynia when the affected area is blown on by a fan

THE PHYSICAL EXAMINATION

- The patient is afebrile
- Obvious vesicular rash in the distribution of the left ophthalmic branch of the trigeminal nerve (V1) (see photo of Renaldo Saldana)
- No auricular lesions bilaterally

OTHER FINDINGS OF NOTE

- Slightly elevated BP
- Normal head, eyes, ears, nose, throat (HEENT) examination
- Normal cardiovascular examination
- Normal pulmonary examination
- Normal abdominal examination
- No peripheral edema
- Normal prostate examination
- No adenopathy

What Tests Would You Like to Order?

The following tests were ordered:
- Complete blood count
- Chemistry profile
- Enzyme-linked immunosorbent assay (ELISA) test for HIV

TEST RESULTS

All testing was within normal limits.

 Clinical Correlation—Putting It All Together

What is the diagnosis?
- Acute herpes zoster of the first division of the trigeminal nerve on the left

The Science Behind the Diagnosis
ANATOMY OF THE TRIGEMINAL NERVE

The trigeminal nerve is the fifth cranial nerve and is denoted by the Roman numeral V. The trigeminal nerve has three divisions and provides sensory innervation for the forehead and eye (V1, ophthalmic), cheek (V2, maxillary), and lower face and jaw (V3, mandibular), as well as motor innervation for the muscles of mastication (Fig. 1.1). The fibers of the trigeminal nerve arise in the trigeminal nerve nucleus, which is the largest of the cranial nerve nuclei. Extending from the midbrain to the upper cervical spinal cord, the trigeminal nerve nucleus is divided into three parts: (1) the mesencephalic trigeminal nucleus, which receives proprioceptive and mechanoreceptor fibers from the mandible and teeth; (2) the main trigeminal nucleus, which receives the majority of the touch and position fibers; and (3) the spinal trigeminal nucleus, which receives pain and temperature fibers.

The sensory fibers of the trigeminal nerve exit the brainstem at the level of the midpons with a smaller motor root emerging from the midpons at the same level. These roots pass in a forward and lateral direction in the posterior cranial fossa across the border of the petrous bone. They then enter a recess called Meckel's cave, which is formed by an invagination of the surrounding dura mater into the middle cranial fossa. The dural pouch that lies just behind the ganglion is called the trigeminal cistern and contains cerebrospinal fluid.

The gasserian ganglion is canoe shaped, with three sensory divisions: (1) the ophthalmic division (V1), which exits the cranium via the superior orbital fissure; (2) the

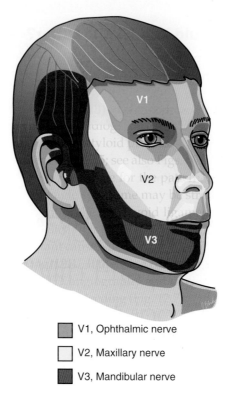

V1, Ophthalmic nerve

V2, Maxillary nerve

V3, Mandibular nerve

Fig. 1.1 The sensory divisions of the trigeminal nerve. (From Waldman S. *Atlas of Interventional Pain Management*. ed. 5. Philadelphia: Elsevier; 2021 [Fig. 12.1].)

maxillary division (V2), which exits the cranium via the foramen rotundum into the pterygopalatine fossa, where it travels anteriorly to enter the infraorbital canal to exit through the infraorbital foramen; and the mandibular division (V3), which exits the cranium via the foramen ovale anterior convex aspect of the ganglion (Fig. 1.2). A small motor root joins the mandibular division as it exits the cranial cavity via the foramen ovale. Three major branches emerge from the trigeminal ganglion (see Fig. 1.2). Each branch innervates a different dermatome. Each branch exits the cranium through a different site. The first division (V1; ophthalmic nerve) exits the cranium through the superior orbital fissure, entering the orbit to innervate the globe and skin in the area above the eye and forehead.

The second division (V2, maxillary nerve) exits through a round hole, the foramen rotundum, into a space posterior to the orbit, the pterygopalatine fossa. It then reenters a canal running inferior to the orbit, the infraorbital canal, and exits through a small hole, the infraorbital foramen, to innervate the skin below the eye and above the mouth. The third division (V3, mandibular nerve) exits the cranium through an oval hole, the foramen ovale. Sensory fibers of the third

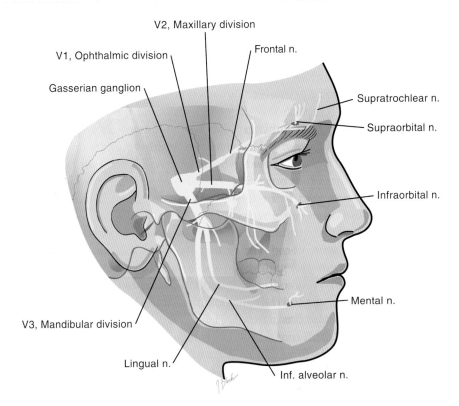

Fig. 1.2 The anatomy of the gasserian ganglion and the branches of the trigeminal nerve. (From Waldman S. *Atlas of Interventional Pain Management*. ed. 5. Philadelphia: Elsevier; 2021 [Fig. 10.2].)

division either travel directly to their target tissues or reenter the mental canal to innervate the teeth, with the terminal branches of this division exiting anteriorly via the mental foramen to provide sensory cutaneous innervation to the skin overlying the mandible.

CLINICAL PRESENTATION

Herpes zoster is an infectious disease caused by the varicella zoster virus (VZV). Primary infection with VZV in a nonimmune host manifests clinically as the childhood disease chickenpox (varicella). Investigators have postulated that during the course of this primary infection, the virus migrates to the dorsal root or cranial ganglia, where it remains dormant and produces no clinically evident disease. In some individuals, the virus reactivates and travels along the sensory pathways of the first division of the trigeminal nerve, where it produces the characteristic pain and skin lesions of herpes zoster, or shingles.

Why reactivation occurs in some individuals but not in others is not fully understood, but investigators have theorized that a decrease in cell-mediated immunity may play an important role in the evolution of this disease by allowing the virus to multiply in the ganglia, spread to the corresponding sensory nerves, and produce clinical disease. Patients who are suffering from malignant disease (particularly lymphoma) or chronic disease and those receiving immunosuppressive therapy (chemotherapy, steroids, radiation) are generally debilitated and thus are much more likely than the healthy population to develop acute herpes zoster (Fig. 1.3). These patients all have in common a decreased cell-mediated immune response, which may also explain why the incidence of shingles increases dramatically in patients older than 60 years and is relatively uncommon in those younger than 20 years.

The first division of the trigeminal nerve is the second most common site for the development of acute herpes zoster after the thoracic dermatomes. Rarely, the virus attacks the geniculate ganglion and results in hearing loss, vesicles in the ear, and pain (Fig. 1.4). This constellation of symptoms is called Ramsay Hunt syndrome and must be distinguished from acute herpes zoster involving the first division of the trigeminal nerve.

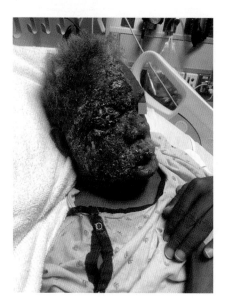

Fig. 1.3 Lateral view of a patient suffering from lymphoma post stem cell transplant with facial lesions includes severe crusting and oozing in a clearly demarcated dermatomal distribution along the right cranial nerve V distribution with associated right facial edema. (From Cheema H, Diedrich A, Kyne B, et al. A case of tri-segmental cranial nerve V herpes zoster. *IDCases*. 2019;18:e00642. ISSN 2214-2509. https://doi.org/10.1016/j.idcr.2019.e00642, http://www.sciencedirect.com/science/article/pii/S2214250919302811 [Fig. 2].)

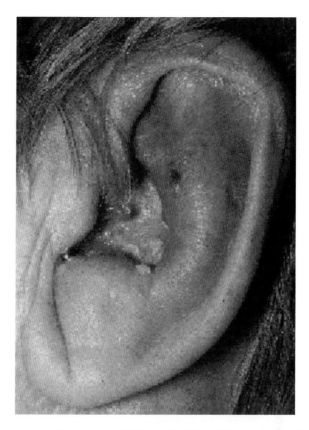

Fig. 1.4 Ramsay Hunt syndrome. (From Waldman S. *Atlas of Common Pain Syndromes*. ed. 4. Philadelphia: Elsevier; 2019 [Fig. 1.1].)

SIGNS AND SYMPTOMS

As viral reactivation occurs, ganglionitis and peripheral neuritis cause pain that may be accompanied by flulike symptoms. The pain generally progresses from a dull, aching sensation to dysesthetic or neuritic pain in the distribution of the first division of the trigeminal nerve. In most patients, the pain of acute herpes zoster precedes the eruption of rash by 3 to 7 days, and this delay often leads to an erroneous diagnosis (see "Differential Diagnosis"). However, in most patients, the clinical diagnosis of shingles is readily made when the characteristic rash appears. As with chickenpox, the rash of herpes zoster appears in crops of macular lesions that rapidly progress to papules and then to vesicles. Eventually, the vesicles coalesce, and crusting occurs (Fig. 1.5). The affected area can be extremely painful, and the pain tends to be exacerbated by any movement or contact (e.g., with clothing or sheets). As the lesions heal, the crust falls away, leaving pink scars that gradually become hypopigmented and atrophic (Fig. 1.6).

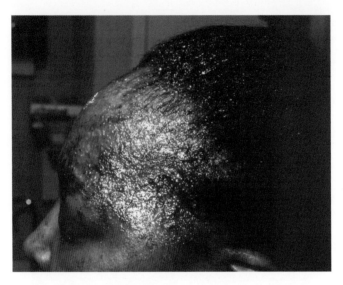

Fig. 1.5 Acute herpes zoster involving the ophthalmic division of the left trigeminal nerve. (From Waldman SD. *Pain management*. Philadelphia: Elsevier; 2007.)

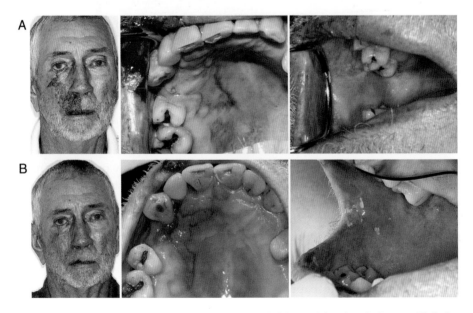

Fig. 1.6 Patient with healing herpes zoster in the second division of the trigeminal nerve. (A) Patient presentation 2 weeks after onset of shingles. (B) Patient presentation 4 weeks after onset of pain. (From Paquin R, Susin L, Welch G, et al. Herpes zoster involving the second division of the trigeminal nerve: case report and literature review. *J Endodont*. 2017;43(9):1569–1573 [Fig. 3].)

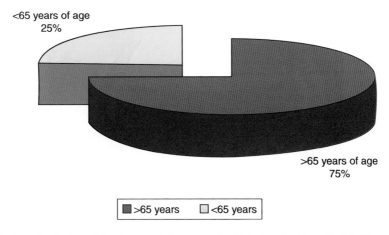

Fig. 1.7 Age of patients suffering from acute herpes zoster. (Data from Waldman S. *Pain Management*. ed. 2. Philadelphia: Saunders; 2011.)

In most patients, the hyperesthesia and pain resolve as the skin lesions heal. In some patients, however, pain persists beyond lesion healing. This common and feared complication of acute herpes zoster is called postherpetic neuralgia, and older persons are affected at a higher rate than the general population suffering from acute herpes zoster (Fig. 1.7). The symptoms of postherpetic neuralgia can vary from a mild, self-limited condition to a debilitating, constantly burning pain that is exacerbated by light touch, movement, anxiety, or temperature change. This unremitting pain may be so severe that it completely devastates the patient's life; ultimately, it can lead to suicide. To avoid this disastrous sequela to a usually benign, self-limited disease, the clinician must use all possible therapeutic efforts in patients with acute herpes zoster of the trigeminal nerve. Ideally, prevention of acute herpes zoster by immunization with Zostrix should be undertaken in all patients 60 years of age and older.

TESTING

Although in most instances the diagnosis is easily made on clinical grounds, confirmatory testing is occasionally required. Such testing may be desirable in patients with other skin lesions that confuse the clinical picture, such as in patients with acquired immunodeficiency syndrome who are suffering from Kaposi sarcoma. In such patients, polymerase chain reaction testing and immunofluorescent antibody testing can rapidly identify herpes zoster virus and distinguish it from herpes simplex infections (Fig. 1.8). In uncomplicated cases, the diagnosis of acute herpes zoster may be strengthened by obtaining a Tzanck smear from the base of a fresh vesicle; this smear reveals multinucleated giant cells and eosinophilic inclusions (Fig. 1.9). However, this inexpensive bedside

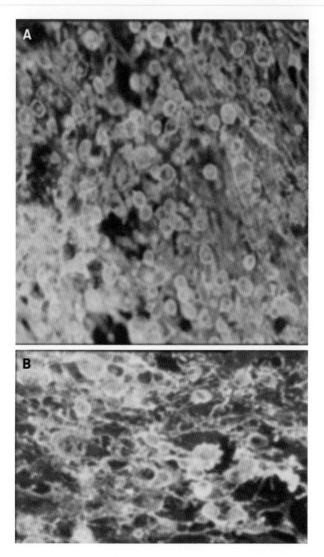

Fig. 1.8 Detection of antivaricella zoster virus immunoglobulin G by the fluorescent antibody to membrane antigen assay. (A) Positive result and (B) negative control. (From Sauerbrei A, Färber I, Brandstädt A, et al. Immunofluorescence test for sensitive detection of varicella-zoster virus-specific IgG: an alternative to fluorescent antibody to membrane antigen test. *J Virol Methods*. 2004;19(1):15–30 [Fig. 1].)

test does not have the ability to distinguish between lesions caused by the VZV and herpes simplex infections.

DIFFERENTIAL DIAGNOSIS

A careful initial evaluation, including a thorough history and physical examination, is indicated in all patients suffering from acute herpes zoster of the

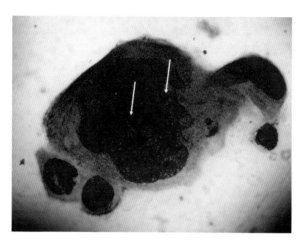

Fig. 1.9 Tzanck smear showing intranuclear inclusion bodies within giant multinucleated cell. May-Grünwald Giemsa stain; original magnification: × 1000. (From Durdu M, Baba M, Seçkin D. The value of Tzanck smear test in diagnosis of erosive, vesicular, bullous, and pustular skin lesions. *J Am Acad Dermatol.* 2008;59(6):958–964 [Fig. 1]. ISSN 0190-9622. https://doi.org/10.1016/j.jaad.2008.07.059, http://www.sciencedirect.com/science/article/pii/S0190962208010669)

trigeminal nerve. The goal is to rule out occult malignant or systemic disease that may be responsible for the patient's immunocompromised state. A prompt diagnosis allows early recognition of changes in clinical status that may presage the development of complications, including myelitis or dissemination of the disease. Other causes of pain in the distribution of the first division of the trigeminal nerve include trigeminal neuralgia, sinus disease, glaucoma, retro-orbital tumor, inflammatory disease (e.g., Tolosa-Hunt syndrome), and intracranial disease, including tumor (Box 1.1).

TREATMENT

The therapeutic challenge in patients presenting with acute herpes zoster of the trigeminal nerve is twofold: (1) the immediate relief of acute pain and symptoms, and (2) the prevention of complications, including postherpetic neuralgia. Most pain specialists agree that the earlier treatment is initiated, the less likely it is that postherpetic neuralgia will develop. Further, because older individuals are at the highest risk for developing postherpetic neuralgia, early and aggressive treatment of this group of patients is mandatory.

Nerve block

Sympathetic neural blockade with local anesthetic and steroid through stellate ganglion block is the treatment of choice to relieve the symptoms of acute herpes

---

BOX 1.1 ■ Causes of Facial Pain

- Trigeminal neuralgia
- Atypical facial pain
- Temporomandibular joint dysfunction
- Temporal arteritis
- Cluster headache
- Autonomic trigeminal cephalgias
- Dental abnormalities
- Acute herpes zoster
- Trauma
- Neoplasm
- Infection
- Diseases of the eye
- Sinus disease
- Inflammatory disorders (e.g., Tolosa-Hunt syndrome)
- Eagle syndrome
- Multiple sclerosis
- Referred pain
- Salivary gland disease
- Vasculitis
- Aneurysms
- Glossopharyngeal neuralia
- Vidian neuralgia
- Psychogenic disorders

---

zoster of the trigeminal nerve, as well as to prevent postherpetic neuralgia. As vesicular crusting occurs, the steroid may also reduce neural scarring. Sympathetic nerve block is thought to achieve these goals by blocking the profound sympathetic stimulation caused by viral inflammation of the nerve and gasserian ganglion. If untreated, this sympathetic hyperactivity can cause ischemia secondary to decreased blood flow of the intraneural capillary bed. If this ischemia is allowed to persist, endoneural edema forms, thus increasing endoneural pressure and causing a further reduction in endoneural blood flow, with irreversible nerve damage.

These sympathetic blocks should be continued aggressively until the patient is pain free and should be reimplemented if the pain returns. Failure to use sympathetic neural blockade immediately and aggressively, especially in older patients, may sentence the patient to a lifetime of suffering from postherpetic neuralgia. Occasionally, some patients do not experience pain relief from stellate ganglion block but do respond to blockade of the trigeminal nerve.

Opioid analgesics

Opioid analgesics can be useful to relieve the aching pain that is common during the acute stages of herpes zoster, while sympathetic nerve blocks are being implemented. Opioids are less effective in relieving neuritic pain, which is also common. Careful administration of potent, long-acting opioid analgesics (e.g., oral morphine elixir, methadone) on a time-contingent rather than an as-needed basis may be a beneficial adjunct to the pain relief provided by sympathetic neural blockade. Because many patients suffering from acute herpes zoster are older or have severe multisystem disease, close monitoring for the potential side effects of potent opioid analgesics (e.g., confusion or dizziness, which may cause a patient to fall) is warranted. Daily dietary fiber supplementation and milk of magnesia should be started along with opioid analgesics to prevent constipation.

Adjuvant analgesics

The anticonvulsant gabapentin represents a first-line treatment for the neuritic pain of acute herpes zoster of the trigeminal nerve. Studies suggest that gabapentin may also help prevent postherpetic neuralgia. Treatment with gabapentin should begin early in the course of the disease; this drug may be used concurrently with neural blockade, opioid analgesics, and other adjuvant analgesics, including antidepressants, if care is taken to avoid central nervous system side effects. Gabapentin is started at a bedtime dose of 300 mg and is titrated upward in 300-mg increments to a maximum of 3600 mg given in divided doses, as side effects allow. Pregabalin represents a reasonable alternative to gabapentin and is better tolerated in some patients. Pregabalin is started at 50 mg three times a day and may be titrated upward to 100 mg three times a day as side effects allow. Because pregabalin is excreted primarily by the kidneys, the dosage should be decreased in patients with compromised renal function.

Carbamazepine should be considered in patients suffering from severe neuritic pain who fail to respond to nerve blocks and gabapentin. If this drug is used, strict monitoring of hematologic parameters is indicated, especially in patients receiving chemotherapy or radiation therapy. Phenytoin may also be beneficial to treat neuritic pain, but it should not be used in patients with lymphoma; the drug may induce a pseudolymphoma-like state that is difficult to distinguish from the actual lymphoma.

Antidepressants may also be useful adjuncts in the initial treatment of patients suffering from acute herpes zoster. On a short-term basis, these drugs help alleviate the significant sleep disturbance that is commonly seen. In addition, antidepressants may be valuable in ameliorating the neuritic component of the pain, which is treated less effectively with opioid analgesics. After several weeks of treatment, antidepressants may exert a mood-elevating effect, which may be desirable in some patients. Care must be taken to observe closely for central nervous system side effects in this patient population. In addition, these drugs may cause urinary retention and constipation, which mistakenly may be attributed to herpes zoster myelitis.

Antiviral agents

A few antiviral agents, including valacyclovir, famciclovir, and acyclovir, can shorten the course of acute herpes zoster and may even help prevent the development of postherpetic neuralgia. They are probably useful in attenuating the disease in immunosuppressed patients. These antiviral agents can be used in conjunction with the aforementioned treatment modalities. Careful monitoring for side effects is mandatory.

Adjunctive treatments

The application of ice packs to the lesions of acute herpes zoster may provide relief in some patients. Application of heat increases pain in most patients, presumably because of the increased conduction of small fibers; however, it is beneficial in an occasional patient and may be worth trying if the application of cold is ineffective. Transcutaneous electrical nerve stimulation and vibration may also be effective in a limited number of patients. The favorable risk-to-benefit ratio of these modalities makes them reasonable alternatives for patients who cannot or will not undergo sympathetic neural blockade or cannot tolerate pharmacologic interventions.

Topical application of aluminum sulfate as a tepid soak provides excellent drying of the crusting and weeping lesions of acute herpes zoster, and most patients find these soaks soothing. Zinc oxide ointment may also be used as a protective agent, especially during the healing phase, when temperature sensitivity is a problem. Disposable diapers can be used as absorbent padding to protect healing lesions from contact with clothing and sheets.

HIGH-YIELD TAKEAWAYS

- The patient is experiencing the acute onset of left forehead pain followed by the appearance of vesicular eruptions in the distribution of the first division of the trigeminal nerve.
- The onset of pain without antecedent trauma followed by the vesicular rash is the classic presentation of acute herpes zoster.
- The rash of acute herpes zoster will follow the distribution of a nerve.
- Immunocompromised states, including old age, predispose the patient to the development of acute herpes zoster.
- Prevention of acute herpes zoster with use of immunization with Zostrix is indicated for patients over the age of 65.
- Aggressive treatment of acute herpes zoster is indicated to avoid the complication of postherpetic neuralgia.

Suggested Readings

Bandaranayake T, Shaw AC. Host resistance and immune aging. *Clin Geriatr Med.* 2016;32(3):415–432.

Corey W, Waldman SD, Waldman RA. Pain of ocular and periocular origin. *Med Clin N Am.* 2013;97(2):293–307. ISSN 0025-7125.

Kansu L, Yilmaz I. Herpes zoster oticus (Ramsay Hunt syndrome) in children: case report and literature review. *Int J Pediatr Otorhinolaryngol.* 2012;76(6):772–776.

Lee HL, Yeo M, Choi GH, et al. Clinical characteristics of headache or facial pain prior to the development of acute herpes zoster of the head. *Clin Neurol Neurosurg.* 2017;152:90–94.

Lee HY, Kim MG, Park DC, et al. Zoster sine herpete causing facial palsy. *Am J Otolaryngol.* 2012;33(5):565–571.

O'Connor KM, Paauw DS. Herpes zoster. *Med Clin North Am.* 2013;97(4):503–522.

Schmader K. Zoster herpes. *Clin Geriatr Med.* 2016;32(3):539–553.

Staikov I, Neykov N, Marinovic B, et al. Herpes zoster as a systemic disease. *Clin Dermatol.* 2014;32(3):424–429.

Yawn BP, Wollan St. PC, Sauver JL, et al. Herpes zoster eye complications: rates and trends. *Mayo Clin Proc.* 2013;88(6):562–570.

Stephanie Ellison

A 32-Year-Old Graphic Designer With Severe Throbbing Left-Sided Headaches

LEARNING OBJECTIVES

- Learn the common types of headache.
- Develop an understanding of clinical presentation of specific headache types.
- Learn to identify prodrome and aura.
- Develop an understanding of the treatment of specific headache types.
- Develop an understanding of the differential diagnosis of headache.
- Develop an understanding of the treatment options for specific headache types.
- Learn how to identify factors that cause concern.

Stephanie Ellison

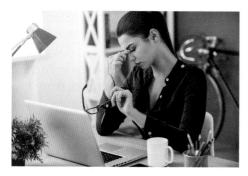

Stephanie Ellison is a 24-year-old graphic designer with the chief complaint of, "My head is throbbing and I'm going to throw up." Stephanie stated that she has had several headaches a month her entire adult life, but over the past several weeks, she has been having debilitating headaches that are getting worse. She said that the headaches have been so bad that she was way behind on her work and that her boyfriend had just about quit speaking to her. I asked Stephanie if she had ever had anything like this before and she said, "I've had headaches since I started my periods, but they seem to have gotten worse since I started working from home. So, I don't know what to do! Nothing makes these headaches better. I know when I am going to get one, but Doctor, once they start, I am just sicker than a dog. All I can do is grab a pan to throw up in and go hide in a dark room." To prove her point, she grabbed the wastebasket next to the examination table and had the dry heaves right there. By the time she finished, tears were running down her face and she closed her eyes and sobbed.

I tried to help Stephanie calm down, and after she tried to vomit a couple more times, I asked her if she had identified anything that triggered her headache and she immediately answered, "My periods." She continued, "I also sometimes get them when my sleep is messed up or when I have the stress of a deadline." I asked her if she was ever woken up with a headache, and she said no, but they often occurred in the morning. "They also got worse when my gynecologist changed my birth control pills because my insurance changed." I asked if anyone else in her family had similar headaches and she said that both her mom and her aunt had the same headaches, but they got better with menopause. I asked if she knew that she was going to get a headache before it actually started and she said, "Absolutely. It's the craziest thing. When I am going to have a headache, it feels like everything looks like it is in a high-definition movie with the subwoofers turned all the way up. I then start to get really sensitive to the light of my computer screen, everything is too loud, and any strong odors make me want to gag. The other crazy thing is that I can't stop yawning. It drives my boyfriend crazy. I just keep yawning over and over again even though I am not tired. Then my vision in my left eye gets all jiggly and shimmery and glittery and I know I am really in trouble. I still don't have any headache, but I know that there is no going back. I've tried all of the usual over-the-counter medications like Excedrin Migraine and those Imitrex shots, but once the eye thing gets going, nothing works to stop the headache." I asked if she had any weakness associated with her headache and she said, "No, just the eye thing, and the nausea and vomiting. I've gotten so dehydrated from the vomiting that I have ended up in the ER a bunch of times. I heard one of the nurses tell the ER doctor that I was a frequent flyer. . .as if I had a choice!" She started crying again. I asked if she experienced smells that nobody else could smell or if she had any difficulty finding words or speaking, and she again said no. "Look, Doctor, I'm not making this stuff up." I told her that I believed her and thought that I had a pretty good idea what was going on.

I asked her what made it better and she said that really nothing worked once the headache got going. Sometimes the shot of demerol and phenergan they gave her in the ER let her go home and sleep the headache off. She started crying and said, "Doctor, what am I going to do? Do you think I have a brain tumor? That's what my boyfriend says!"

I asked Stephanie to use one finger to point at the spot where it hurt the most. She pointed to her left temple. I asked her what the pain was like—an ache, sharp, stabbing, burning—and she immediately said, "throbbing." I asked whether the headache was on both sides or just one side, and she immediately answered, "It's always on my left side." I asked Stephanie from the time that she knew that she was going to get the headache until the time it was at its worst, was it a period of seconds, minutes, or hours, and she said, "It is always at least a couple of hours before it's the worst."

I asked Stephanie if I could examine her and she said, "You can pull out a couple of toenails if you can get rid of my headaches." I smiled and said that I hoped that would not be necessary. On physical examination, Stephanie was afebrile. Her respirations were 16 and her pulse was 84 and regular. Her blood pressure was 126/80. There were no cranial abnormalities, and her ears and throat were normal. When I grabbed my ophthalmoscope to examine Stephanie's eyes, she asked in a weak voice, "Do you have to shine that light in my eyes? I am really sensitive to light with my headaches." I told her I would be as quick as I could, but that I really need to check things out. Her pupils were round, equal, and reactive to light. It took a little effort to perform a fundoscopic examination because Stephanie kept pulling away from the light. I reassured her and was happy to note that there was no papilledema. Her cardiopulmonary examination was normal, as was her thyroid. Her abdominal examination revealed no abnormal mass or organomegaly, but she was a little tender to palpation from all the vomiting. No rebound tenderness was present. There was no costovertebral angle (CVA) tenderness. There was no peripheral edema. A careful neurologic examination of the upper and lower extremities revealed there was no evidence of weakness, lack of coordination, or peripheral or entrapment neuropathy, and her deep tendon reflexes were normal. Stephanie's mental status exam was within normal limits.

Key Clinical Points—What's Important and What's Not

THE HISTORY

- Episodic headaches entire adult life
- Headaches are unilateral
- Character of pain of the headaches is throbbing in nature
- Headaches are preceded by a prodrome consisting of changes in the quality of vision and hearing and aversion to strong odors, as well as persistent yawning
- Patient experiences a painless prodrome consisting of visual disturbance and photophobia
- Patient denies olfactory aura, weakness, or speech difficulties
- No fever or chills
- Notes significant nausea and vomiting associated with the onset of pain
- Significant disability associated with headaches
- Headaches associated with menstruation

THE PHYSICAL EXAMINATION

- Patient is afebrile
- Normal fundoscopic exam
- Examination of the cranium is normal
- Neurologic exam is normal other than photophobia
- Frequent vomiting during examination

OTHER FINDINGS OF NOTE

- Normal cardiovascular examination
- Normal pulmonary examination
- Normal abdominal examination
- No peripheral edema
- Normal upper and lower extremity neurologic examination, motor and sensory examination

 What Tests Would You Like to Order?

The following test was ordered:
- Magnetic resonance imaging (MRI) of the brain

TEST RESULTS

The MRI of the brain was normal.

📋 Clinical Correlation—Putting It All Together

What is the diagnosis?
Migraine with aura

The Science Behind the Diagnosis

CLINICAL SYNDROME

Migraine headache is a periodic unilateral headache that may begin in childhood but almost always develops before age 30 years. Attacks occur with variable frequency, ranging from every few days to once every several months. More frequent migraine headaches are often associated with a phenomenon called analgesic rebound. Between 60% and 70% of patients who suffer from migraine are female, and many report a family history of migraine headache. The personality type of migraineurs has been described as meticulous, neat, compulsive, and often rigid. They tend to be obsessive in their daily routines and often find it hard to cope with the stresses of everyday life. Migraine headache may be triggered by changes in sleep patterns or diet or by the ingestion of tyramine-containing foods, monosodium glutamate, nitrates, chocolate, wine, or citrus fruits. Changes in endogenous and exogenous hormones, such as with the use of birth control pills, can also trigger migraine headache, as can the ingestion of nitroglycerine for angina. The typical migraine headache is characterized by four phases: (1) the prodrome, (2) the aura, (3) the headache, and (4) the postdrome (Fig. 2.1). Some migraineurs will experience a premonition or warning that a migraine may be on the horizon. This premonition or warning is known as a prodrome and may manifest as mood

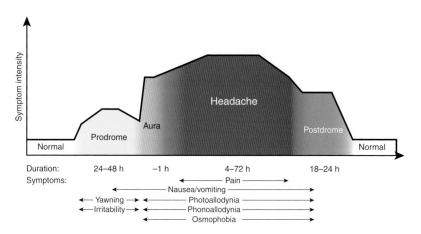

Fig. 2.1 The four phases of migraine. (Redrawn from Burgos-Vega C, Moy J, Dussor G. Meningeal afferent signaling and the pathophysiology of migraine. *Prog Mol Biol Transl Sci.* 2015;131:537–564.)

changes, food cravings, frequent yawning, changes in libido, and constipation. Approximately 20% of patients suffering from migraine headache also experience a neurologic event called an aura before the onset of pain. The aura most often takes the form of a visual disturbance, but it may also manifest as an alteration in smell or hearing; these are called olfactory and auditory auras, respectively. Following a migraine headache, some patients will experience a period of confusion, dizziness, weakness, or elation known as a postdrome. While the exact pathophysiology of migraine has not been elucidated, it appears that that the symptoms and pain associated with migraine headache are the result of functional abnormalities in multiple parts of the central nervous system, as depicted in Fig. 2.2. Other factors, including migraine-associated genes, hormones, environment, stress, and neuroendocrine function may also play a role (Fig. 2.3).

SIGNS AND SYMPTOMS

Migraine headache is, by definition, a unilateral headache. Although the headache may change sides with each episode, the headache is never bilateral at its onset. The pain of migraine headache is usually periorbital or retro-orbital. It is pounding, and its intensity is severe. The time from onset to peak of migraine pain is short, ranging from 20 minutes to 1 hour. In contradistinction from tension-type headache, migraine headache is often associated with systemic symptoms, including nausea and vomiting, photophobia, and sonophobia, as well as alterations in appetite, mood, and libido. Menstruation is a common trigger of migraine headache.

As mentioned, in approximately 20% of patients, migraine headache is preceded by an aura (called migraine with aura). The aura is thought to be the result of ischemia of specific regions of the cerebral cortex. A visual aura often occurs 30 to 60 minutes before the onset of headache pain; this may take the form of blind spots, called scotoma, scintillation, or a zigzag disruption of the visual field, called fortification spectrum (Figs. 2.4 and 2.5). Occasionally, patients with migraine lose an entire visual field during the aura. Auditory auras usually take the form of hypersensitivity to sound, but other alterations of hearing, such as sounds perceived as farther away than they actually are, have also been reported. Olfactory auras may take the form of strong odors of substances that are not actually present or extreme hypersensitivity to otherwise normal odors, such as coffee or copy machine toner. Migraine that manifests without other neurologic symptoms is called migraine without aura.

Rarely, patients who suffer from migraine experience prolonged neurologic dysfunction associated with the headache pain. Such neurologic dysfunction may last for more than 24 hours and is termed migraine with prolonged aura. These patients are at risk for the development of permanent neurologic deficit, and risk factors such as hypertension, smoking, and oral contraceptives must be addressed. Even less common than migraine with prolonged aura is migraine

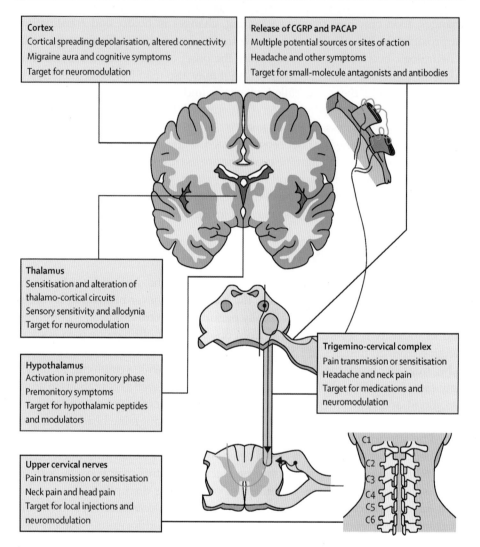

Cortex
Cortical spreading depolarisation, altered connectivity
Migraine aura and cognitive symptoms
Target for neuromodulation

Release of CGRP and PACAP
Multiple potential sources or sites of action
Headache and other symptoms
Target for small-molecule antagonists and antibodies

Thalamus
Sensitisation and alteration of
thalamo-cortical circuits
Sensory sensitivity and allodynia
Target for neuromodulation

Hypothalamus
Activation in premonitory phase
Premonitory symptoms
Target for hypothalamic peptides
and modulators

Trigemino-cervical complex
Pain transmission or sensitisation
Headache and neck pain
Target for medications and
neuromodulation

Upper cervical nerves
Pain transmission or sensitisation
Neck pain and head pain
Target for local injections and
neuromodulation

C1
C2
C3
C4
C5
C6

Fig. 2.2 Migraine involves the simultaneous alteration in function of multiple components of the central nervous and peripheral nervous systems, some of which are represented in this diagram. Each of these components could be responsible for different symptoms of migraine, and each could represent a specific therapeutic target in individual patients. Red arrows indicate sensory inputs from the trigeminal nerve and upper cervical nerve roots, which converge in the trigeminocervical complex. CGRP, Calcitonin gene–related peptide; PACAP, pituitary adenylate cyclase-activating polypeptide. (Reprinted with permission from Elsevier (From Charles A. The pathophysiology of migraine: implications for clinical management. *Lancet Neurol.* 2018;17(2):174–182 [Fig. 2]. ISSN 1474-4422).)

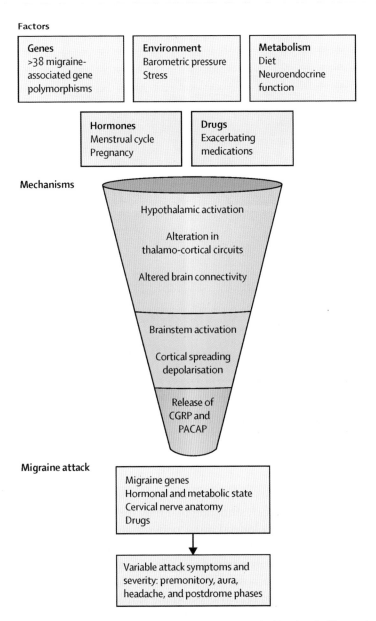

Fig. 2.3 Contributing factors and mechanisms of a migraine attack. (Reprinted with permission from Elsevier (From Charles, A., The pathophysiology of migraine: implications for clinical management, *Lancet Neurol.* 2018;17(2):174–182 [Fig. 2].))

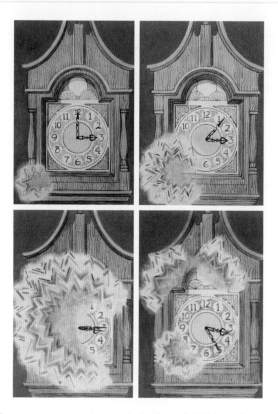

Fig. 2.4   The migraine aura represented as a clock. *Top left:* Initial small paracentral scotoma; *top right:* enlarging scotoma 7 minutes later; *bottom left:* scotoma obscuring much of central vision 15 minutes later; *bottom right:* break-up of scotoma at 20 minutes. (From S.L. Hupp, L.B. Kline, J.J. Corbett. Visual disturbances of migraine. *Surv Ophthalmol*, 33 (1989), pp. 221–236.)

with complex aura. Patients suffering from migraine with complex aura experience significant neurologic dysfunction that may include aphasia or hemiplegia. As with migraine with prolonged aura, patients suffering from migraine with complex aura may develop permanent neurologic deficits.

Patients suffering from all forms of migraine headache appear systemically ill (Fig. 2.6). Pallor, tremulousness, diaphoresis, and light sensitivity are common physical findings. The temporal artery and the surrounding area may be tender. If an aura is present, results of the neurologic examination will be abnormal; the neurologic examination is usually within normal limits before, during, and after migraine without aura.

TESTING

No specific test exists for migraine headache. Testing is aimed primarily at identifying occult pathologic processes or other diseases that may mimic migraine

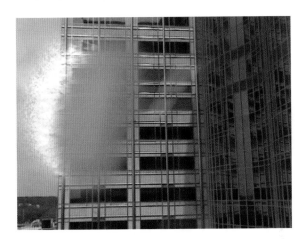

Fig. 2.5 A representation of the positive (scintillation) and negative (relative scotoma) symptoms that can occur during attacks of typical migraine visual aura. (From Foroozan R, Cutrer FM. Transient neurologic dysfunction in migraine. *Neurol Clin.* 2019;37(4):673–694 [Fig. 3]. ISSN 0733-8619, ISBN 9780323708708, https://doi.org/10.1016/j.ncl.2019.06.002, http://www.sciencedirect.com/science/article/pii/S0733861919300593)

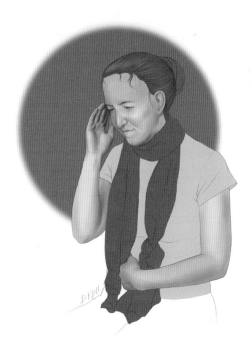

Fig. 2.6 Migraine headache is an episodic, unilateral headache that occurs most commonly in female patients. The patient will often appear systemically ill. (From Waldman S. *Atlas of Common Pain Syndromes.* ed. 4. Philadelphia: Elsevier; 2019 [Fig. 2-3].)

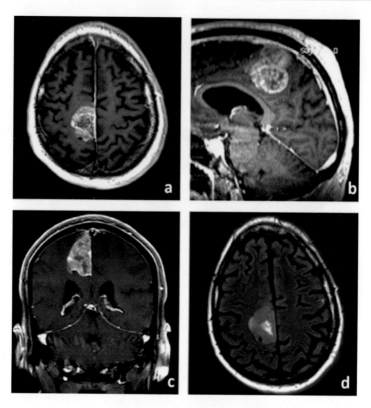

Fig. 2.7 Magnetic resonance imaging (MRI) of the brain is indicated in all patients who present with migraine headache. MRI of the brain in a patient who presented with a chief complaint of headache. (a) Axial T1 MRI after administration of gadolinium contrast demonstrating a right frontoparietal lesion with heterogeneous enhancement. (b) Sagittal T1 with contrast. (c) Coronal T1 with contrast. The broad dural attachment to the falx is well visualized. (d) Axial T2 fluid attenuated inversion recovery (FLAIR) sequence demonstrates a small amount of surrounding edema. (From Michaelson NM, Connerney M. Glioblastoma multiforme that unusually present with radiographic dural tails: questioning the diagnostic paradigm with a rare case report. *Radiol Case Rep*. 2020;15(7):1087–1090 [Fig. 1]. ISSN 1930-0433, https://doi.org/10.1016/j.radcr.2020.05.007, http://www.sciencedirect.com/science/article/pii/S1930043320301771)

headache (see "Differential Diagnosis"). All patients with a recent onset of headache thought to be migraine should undergo MRI of the brain (Fig. 2.7). If neurologic dysfunction accompanies the patient's headache symptoms, MRI should be performed with and without gadolinium contrast medium; magnetic resonance angiography should be considered as well. MRI should also be performed in patients with previously stable migraine headaches who experience an inexplicable change in symptoms. Screening laboratory tests, including an erythrocyte sedimentation rate, complete blood count, and automated blood chemistry, should be performed if the diagnosis of migraine is in question. Fundoscopic examination is indicated in all patients presenting with headache (Fig. 2.8).

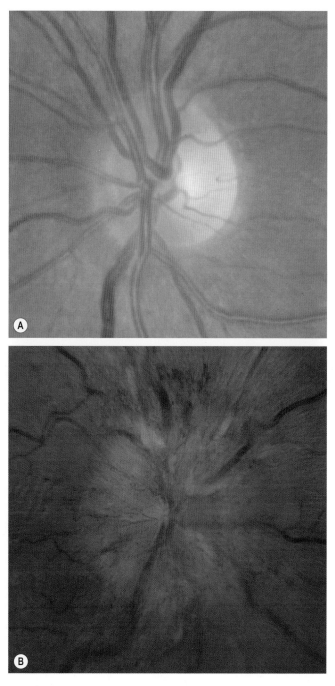

Fig. 2.8   (A) Normal optic disc. Disc swelling associated with (B) elevated intracranial pressure (papille-dema), (C) anterior ischemic optic neuropathy, and (D) optic neuritis. (From Liu G, Volpe N, Galetta S, et al. *Galetta's Neuro-Ophthalmology*. ed. 3. Philadelphia: Elsevier; 2019:197−235 [Fig. 6-1a-d]. ISBN 9780323340441, https://doi.org/10.1016/B978-0-323-34044-1.00006-7, http://www.sciencedirect.com/science/article/pii/B9780323340441000067)

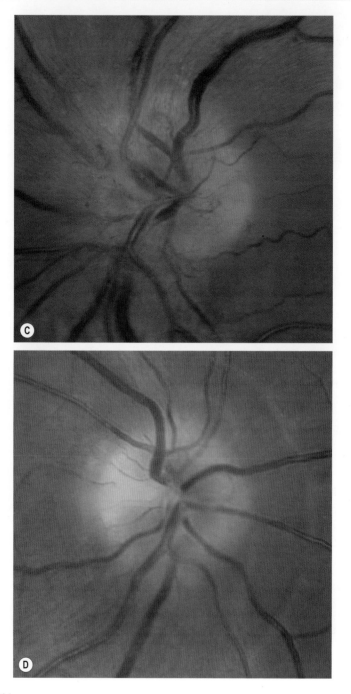

Fig. 2.8, cont'd.

Ophthalmologic evaluation is indicated in all patients who experience significant ocular symptoms associated with their headache symptomatology.

DIFFERENTIAL DIAGNOSIS

The diagnosis of migraine headache is usually made on clinical grounds by obtaining a targeted headache history. Tension-type headache is often confused with migraine headache, and this misdiagnosis can lead to illogical treatment plans because these two headache syndromes are managed quite differently. Table 2.1 distinguishes migraine headache from tension-type headache and should help clarify the diagnosis.

Diseases of the eyes, ears, nose, and sinuses may also mimic migraine headache. The targeted history and physical examination, combined with appropriate testing, should allow the clinician to identify and properly treat any underlying diseases of these organ systems. Many conditions may mimic migraine and must be considered when treating patients with headache. These include glaucoma, temporal arteritis, sinusitis, intracranial disease (including chronic subdural hematoma, tumor brain abscess, hydrocephalus, and pseudotumor cerebri), and inflammatory conditions (including sarcoidosis and Tolosa-Hunt syndrome) (Table 2.2). Because many of the things that mimic migraine can be life-threatening, the clinician should remain vigilant for signs or symptoms that are red flags (Table 2.3).

TREATMENT

When deciding how best to treat a patient suffering from migraine, the clinician should consider the frequency and severity of the headaches, their effect on the patient's lifestyle, the presence of focal or prolonged neurologic disturbances, the results of previous testing and treatment, any history of previous drug abuse or misuse, and the presence of other systemic diseases (e.g., peripheral vascular

TABLE 2.1 ■ Comparison of Migraine Headache and Tension-Type Headache

	Migraine Headache	Tension-Type Headache
Onset-to-peak interval	Minutes to 1 hr	Hours to days
Frequency	Rarely >1/wk	Often daily or continuous
Location	Temporal	Nuchal or circumferential
Character	Pounding	Aching, pressure, bandlike
Laterality	Always unilateral	Usually bilateral
Aura	May be present	Never present
Nausea and vomiting	Common	Rare
Duration	Usually <24 hr	Often days

TABLE 2.2 ■ Differential Diagnosis Of Migraine Headache

Primary Headache Disorders
- Trigeminal autonomic cephalalgias
  - Cluster headache
  - Paroxysmal hemicranias
  - Hemicrania continua
  - Short-lasting unilateral neuralgiform headache attacks (SUNCT/SUNA)
- Hypnic headache
- New daily persistent headache

Secondary Headache Disorders
- Medication overuse headaches
  - Analgesic rebound headache
- Vascular headaches
  - Cerebral aneurysms
  - Arterial dissection
  - Temporal arteritis
  - Intracranial hemorrhage
  - Stroke
  - Venous sinus thrombosis
  - Transient ischemic attack
  - Reversible vasoconstriction syndrome
  - Vasculitis
  - Thunderclap headache
- Headaches associated with neoplasm
- Headaches associated with infection
  - Sinusitis
  - Meningitis
  - Dental infections
  - Lyme disease
  - Herpes simplex encephalitis
- Headaches associated with abnormalities of cerebrospinal fluid pressure
  - Idiopathic intracranial hypertension
  - Low pressure cerebrospinal fluid headaches
    - Spontaneous leaks
    - Postdural puncture headache
- Headaches associated with medications
  - Nitroglycerine
  - Caffeine withdrawal
  - Antihypertensives
  - Erectile dysfunction medications
  - Hormones, including oral contraceptives
- Headaches associated with systemic disease
  - Hypertension
  - Epilepsy
  - Hypothyroidism
  - Hypoglycemia
  - Renal failure
  - Sacroidosis
  - Tolosa-Hunt syndrome
- Headaches associated with exposure to toxins
  - Carbon monoxide poisoning
  - Hydrocarbon exposure
  - Nitroglycerin

TABLE 2.3 ■ Red Flags in the Patient With Headache

- First or worst headache
- Headache associated with fever, stiff neck, or systemic disease
- Headaches with a rapid onset to peak
- Headaches precipitated by Valsalva maneuver
- Headaches associated with neurologic signs or symptoms
- A change in the clinical features of a previously stable headache
- Headaches associated with head injury or major trauma
- Headaches with atypical presentation
- Headaches that fail to respond to appropriate optimized therapy

or coronary artery disease) that may preclude the use of certain treatment modalities.

If the patient's migraine headaches occur infrequently, a trial of abortive therapy may be warranted. However, if the headaches occur with greater frequency or cause the patient to miss work or be hospitalized, prophylactic therapy is warranted.

Abortive therapy

For abortive therapy to be effective, it must be initiated at the first sign of headache. This is often difficult because of the short interval between the onset and peak of migraine headache, coupled with the problem that migraine sufferers often experience nausea and vomiting that may limit the use of oral medications. By altering the route of administration to parenteral or transmucosal, this situation can be avoided.

Abortive medications that can be considered in patients with migraine headache include compounds that contain isometheptene mucate (e.g., Midrin), the nonsteroidal antiinflammatory drug (NSAID) naproxen, ergot alkaloids, the triptans (including sumatriptan, rizatriptan, almotriptan, naratriptan, zolmitriptan, frovatriptan, and eletriptan), and intravenous lidocaine combined with antiemetic compounds. Recent clinical experience suggests that the calcitonin gene—related peptide receptor antagonist, ubrogepant, may represent a safe alternative to other abortive therapies without many of the side effects and risks. The inhalation of 100% oxygen may abort migraine headache, and sphenopalatine ganglion block with local anesthetic may be effective. Caffeine-containing preparations, barbiturates, ergotamines, triptans, and opioids have a propensity to cause a phenomenon called analgesic rebound headache, which may ultimately be more difficult to treat than the original migraine. The ergotamines and triptans should not be used in patients with coexistent peripheral vascular disease, coronary artery disease, or hypertension. Anecdotal reports suggest that cannabis may provide symptom relief in some headache sufferers.

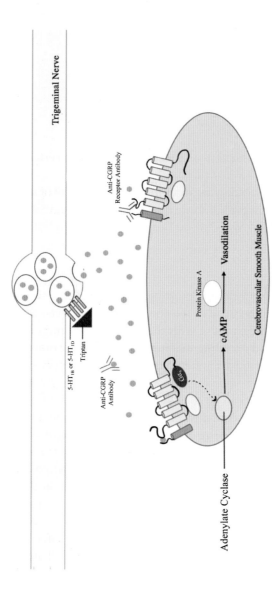

Fig. 2.9 Mechanisms of action of triptans and monoclonal antibodies targeting the calcitonin gene–related peptide (CGRP) or the CGRP receptor. CGRP is released from the trigeminal nerve to activate its receptor. Activating this receptor leads to relaxation of smooth muscles, including those of the vasculature, which results in vasodilation of blood vessels. The new monoclonal antibodies target either CGRP or the CGRP receptors. The anti-CGRP antibodies, fremane-zumab and galcanezumab, bind directly to CGRP after it is released from the trigeminal nerve. Erenumab, the anti-CGRP receptor antibody, binds directly to the CGRP receptor, which blocks the CGRP molecule binding. Triptans work through a different mechanism of action by blocking 5-HT₁B or 5-HT₁D. (From Spindler B, Ryan M. Medications approved for preventing migraine headaches. *Am J Med.* 2020;133(6):664–667 [Fig. 1]. ISSN 0002-9343, https://doi.org/10.1016/j.amjmed.2020.01.031, http://www.sciencedirect.com/science/article/pii/S0002934320301431)

Prophylactic therapy

For most patients with migraine headache, prophylactic therapy is a better option than abortive therapy. The mainstay of prophylactic therapy is beta-blocking agents. Propranolol, metoprolol, timolol, and most other drugs in this class can control or decrease the frequency and intensity of migraine headache and help prevent auras. An 80-mg daily dose of the long-acting formulation is a reasonable starting point for most patients with migraine. Propranolol should not be used in patients with asthma or other reactive airway diseases.

Valproic acid, calcium channel blockers (e.g., verapamil), clonidine, tricyclic antidepressants, the angiotensin-converting enzyme inhibitor lisinopril, and NSAIDs have also been used for the prophylaxis of migraine headache. Onabotulinum toxin A may also provide migraine prophylaxis in selected patients. A new group of humanized monoclonal antibodies that target calcitonin gene-related peptide (CGRP)—erenumab, fremanezumab, and galcanezumab—have been approved by the Food and Drug Administration for migraine prophylaxis (Fig. 2.9). Each of these drugs has advantages and disadvantages, and the clinician should tailor a treatment plan that best meets the needs of the individual patient.

COMPLICATIONS AND PITFALLS

In most patients, migraine headache is a painful but not life-threatening disease. However, patients who suffer from migraine with prolonged aura or migraine with complex aura are at risk for the development of permanent neurologic deficits. Such patients are best treated by headache specialists who are familiar with these unique risks and are better equipped to deal with them. Occasionally, prolonged nausea and vomiting associated with severe migraine headache may result in dehydration that necessitates hospitalization and treatment with intravenous fluids.

HIGH-YIELD TAKEAWAYS

- The patient is afebrile, making an acute infectious etiology unlikely.
- The patient's headaches are unilateral.
- The character of the patient's headache pain is throbbing.
- The patient experiences a prodrome as part of her headache pattern.
- The patient experiences an aura as part of her headache pattern.
- The patient does not experience other neurologic symptoms such as weakness or speech disturbance associated with her headaches.

(Continued)

- The patient has significant photophobia and nausea and vomiting associated with her headaches.
- The patient is experiencing significant disability associated with her headaches.
- The patient experiences headache with menstruation.
- The patient is on oral contraceptives.
- The patient's MRI is negative.
- There are no red flags.

Suggested Readings

Charles A. The pathophysiology of migraine: implications for clinical management. *Lancet Neurol*. 2018;17(2):174−182.

Cuttler C, Spradlin A, Cleveland MJ, et al. Short- and long-term effects of cannabis on headache and migraine. *J Pain*. 2020;21(5−6):722−730.

Evans RW. Diagnostic testing for migraine and other primary headaches. *Neurol Clin*. 2019;37(4):707−725.

Finkel AG. Botulinum toxin and the treatment of headache: a clinical review. *Toxicon*. 2015;107(Pt A):114−119.

Hale N, Paauw DS. Diagnosis and treatment of headache in the ambulatory care setting: a review of classic presentations and new considerations in diagnosis and management. *Med Clin North Am*. 2014;98(3):505−527.

Peck KR, Johnson YL, Smitherman TA, et al., eds. *Handbook of Clinical Neurology*. Philadelphia: Elsevier; 2016:283−293. [vol 138].

Spindler BL, Ryan M. Medications approved for preventing migraine headaches. *Am J Med*. 2020;133(6):664−667.

Waldman SD. *Migraine headache. Atlas of Common Pain Syndromes*. 4th ed. Philadelphia: Elsevier; 2019:6−9.

Waldman SD. *Migraine headache. Pain Review*. ed. 2. Philadelphia: Elsevier; 2016: 200−203.

Younger DS. Epidemiology of migraine. *Neurol Clin*. 2020;34(4):849−861.

Abby Austin

A 30-Year-Old Administrative Assistant With Frequent Headaches Involving the Head and Neck

LEARNING OBJECTIVES

- Learn the common types of headache.
- Understand the difference between primary and secondary headaches.
- Develop an understanding of clinical presentation of specific headache types.
- Develop an understanding of the treatment of specific headache types.
- Develop an understanding of the differential diagnosis of headache.
- Learn how to identify factors that cause concern.

Abby Austin

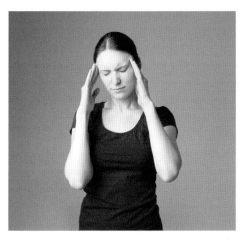

Abby Austin is a 30-year-old administrative assistant with the chief complaint of, "It feels like my head is in a vise." Abby explained that she couldn't remember the last time she didn't have a headache. "It seems like I wake up with the headache and by the end of the day, there it is. It feels like I've been wearing a headband that is too tight, like there is a band around my temples and the back of my head. After spending the day dealing with my crazy micromanager of a boss, my neck muscles are just killing me, and I just want to get out of there and chill!"

Abby said that most days she had headaches, and that while they never kept her from going to work, she just felt worn out from them. "Doctor, my sleep is really messed up. I keep waking up around 4 AM with a headache brewing and I just can't get back to sleep. I go ahead and get up, but by the end of the day, I feel pretty rough."

I asked Abby how long she suffered from headaches and she said, "I've had headaches about as long as I can remember. My mom always had headaches, and I can remember her making my brother and me go outside and play because we were making her headache worse." Abby denied any nausea, vomiting, or other neurologic symptoms associated with her headaches. She said, "By the end of the day, the brightness of my computer monitor seems to aggravate the headache, and I really just want my boss to shut up, but other than the tightness around my head and neck ache, I don't have any other symptoms with my headaches."

I asked Abby if she had identified anything that triggered her headache and she immediately answered, "My boss. I just can't take the stress anymore." I asked Abby if she knew whether she was going to get a headache before the headache actually started, and she said, "Not really." She continued, "Often I wake up with a headache in the making, but it is just there. There are not really any warning signs." I asked about her neck and she said, "By the end of the day, I just want someone to give me a neck massage. I thought it was my pillow, so I bought a MyPillow, and it only made it worse. I feel like the neck and headaches are one and the same."

I asked her what made it better and she said, "I've tried all of the usual over-the-counter medications like Excedrin Migraine and Advil, but they really upset my stomach, so I can't take them very often. A heating pad and a neck massage seems to help a little."

I asked Abby to use one finger to point at the spot where it hurt the most, and she pointed to both her temples and then started rubbing her neck. I asked her what the pain was like: an ache, sharp, stabbing, burning. She immediately said, "It's like my head is being squeezed in a vise. No throbbing, just a squeezing, achy feeling." I asked whether the headache was on both sides or just one side, and she said it was always on both sides and in her neck. I asked Abby from the time that she knew she was going to get the headache until the time it was at its worst, whether it was a period of seconds, minutes, or hours. She said, "It is always at least hours to a day before it is at its worst."

I asked Abby if I could examine her and she said, "That's why I'm here. I just have to get rid of these headaches." On physical examination, Abby was afebrile. Her respirations were 16 and her pulse was 78 and regular. Her blood pressure was 126/80. There were no cranial abnormalities and her head, eyes, ears, nose, throat (HEENT) examination was completely normal, as was her fundoscopic examination. Her cervical paraspinous muscles were tender to deep palpation, but no myofascial trigger points were identified. Her cardiopulmonary examination was normal, as was her thyroid. Her abdominal examination revealed no abnormal mass or organomegaly, and no rebound tenderness was present. There was no costovertebral angle (CVA) tenderness. There was no peripheral edema. A careful neurologic examination of the upper and lower extremities revealed there was no evidence of weakness, lack of coordination, or peripheral or entrapment neuropathy, and her deep tendon reflexes were normal. Abby's mental status exam was within normal limits.

Key Clinical Points—What's Important and What's Not
THE HISTORY

- Episodic headaches entire adult life
- Headaches are bilateral
- Headaches are bitemporal with bandlike tightness
- Headaches are associated with nuchal pain
- Character of pain of the headaches is aching in nature, without throbbing
- No prodrome or aura
- Significant sleep disturbance
- No fever or chills
- Patient denies significant nausea and vomiting associated with the headache
- Minimal disability associated with headaches
- Headaches associated with work stress

THE PHYSICAL EXAMINATION

- Patient is afebrile
- Normal fundoscopic exam
- Examination of the cranium is normal
- Neurologic exam is normal
- Tenderness of the paraspinous muscles without myofascial trigger points

OTHER FINDINGS OF NOTE

- Normal cardiovascular examination
- Normal pulmonary examination
- Normal abdominal examination
- No peripheral edema
- Normal upper and lower extremity neurologic examination, motor and sensory examination

 What Tests Would You Like to Order?

The following test was ordered:
- Magnetic resonance imaging (MRI) of the brain

TEST RESULTS

The MRI of the brain was normal.

 Clinical Correlation—Putting It All Together

What is the diagnosis?
Tension-type headache

The Science Behind the Diagnosis
CLINICAL SYNDROME

Tension-type headache, formerly known as muscle contraction headache, is the most common type of headache that afflicts humankind. It can be episodic or chronic, and it may or may not be related to muscle contraction. Significant sleep disturbance usually occurs. Patients with tension-type headache are often characterized as having multiple unresolved conflicts surrounding work, marriage, and social relationships, and psychosexual difficulties. Testing with the Minnesota Multiphasic Personality Inventory in large groups of patients with tension-type headache revealed not only borderline depression but somatization as well. Most researchers believe that this somatization takes the form of abnormal muscle contraction in some patients; in others, it results in simple headache.

SIGNS AND SYMPTOMS

Tension-type headache is usually bilateral, but it can be unilateral; it often involves the frontotemporal, and occipital regions (Fig. 3.1). It may present as a bandlike, nonpulsatile ache or tightness in the aforementioned anatomic areas (Fig. 3.2). Associated neck symptoms are common. Tension-type headache evolves over a period of hours or days and then tends to remain constant, without progression. It has no associated aura, but significant sleep disturbance is usually present. This disturbance may manifest as difficulty falling asleep, frequent awakening at night, or early awakening. These headaches most frequently occur between 4 and 8 AM and 4 and 8 PM. Although both sexes are affected, female patients predominate. No hereditary pattern to tension-type headache is found, but this type of headache may occur in family clusters because children mimic and learn the pain behavior of their parents.

The triggering event for acute, episodic tension-type headache is invariably either physical or psychological stress. This may take the form of a fight with a

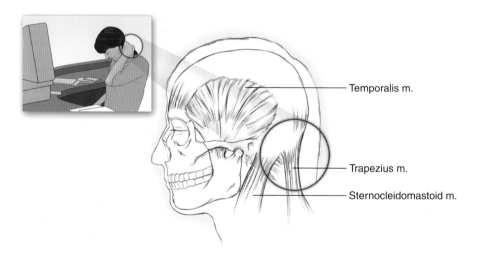

Fig. 3.1 Tension-type headache is almost always bilateral and involves the frontotemporal, and occipital regions. Mental or physical stress is often the precipitating factor in tension-type headache. *m.*, Muscle. (From Waldman S. *Atlas of Common Pain Syndromes*. ed. 4. Philadelphia: Elsevier; 2019 [Fig. 3.1].)

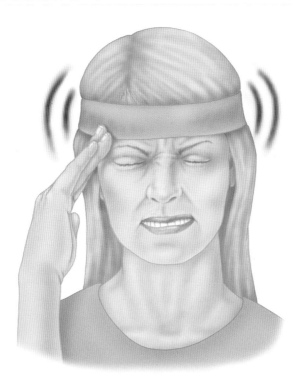

Fig. 3.2 Tension-type headache presents as a bandlike, nonpulsatile ache or tightness in the fore-head, temples, neck, and occipital region. (Redrawn from Kaufman DM. Kaufman's clinical neurology for psychiatrists. 7th ed. Philadelphia: Elsevier; 2013:F9-1.)

coworker or spouse or an exceptionally heavy workload. Physical stress, such as a long drive, working with the neck in a strained position, acute cervical spine injury resulting from whiplash, or prolonged exposure to the glare from computer monitors and mobile devices, may precipitate a headache. A worsening of preexisting degenerative cervical spine conditions, such as cervical spondylosis, can also trigger a tension-type headache. The pathologic process responsible for the development of tension-type headache can produce temporomandibular joint dysfunction as well.

TESTING

No specific test exists for tension-type headache. Testing is aimed primarily at identifying an occult pathologic process or other diseases that may mimic tension-type headache (see "Differential Diagnosis"). All patients with a recent onset of headache that is thought to be tension type should undergo MRI of the brain and, if significant occipital or nuchal symptoms are present, of the cervical spine. MRI should also be performed in patients with previously stable tension-

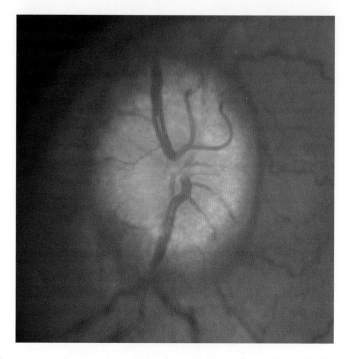

Fig. 3.3 Champagne-cork appearance of chronic papilledema. The whitish, glistening areas on the optic disc head represent gliosis and extruded axoplasm. Note the conspicuous absence of peripapillary hemorrhages. (From Liu G, Volpe N, Galetta S, et al. *Galetta's Neuro-Ophthalmology.* ed. 3. Philadelphia: Elsevier; 2019:197–235 [Fig. 6.7].)

type headaches who have experienced a recent change in symptoms. Screening laboratory tests consisting of a complete blood count, erythrocyte sedimentation rate, and automated blood chemistry should be performed if the diagnosis of tension-type headache is in question. Fundoscopic examination is indicated in all patients presenting with headache (Fig. 3.3). Ophthalmologic evaluation is indicated in all patients who experience significant ocular symptoms associated with their headache symptomatology.

DIFFERENTIAL DIAGNOSIS

Tension-type headache is usually diagnosed on clinical grounds by obtaining a targeted headache history. Despite their obvious differences, tension-type headache is often incorrectly diagnosed as migraine headache. Such misdiagnosis can lead to illogical treatment plans and poor control of headache symptoms. Table 3.1 helps distinguish tension-type headache from migraine headache and should aid the clinician in making the correct diagnosis.

TABLE 3.1 ■ Comparison of Tension-Type Headache and Migraine Headache

	Tension-Type Headache	Migraine Headache
Onset-to-peak interval	Hours to days	Minutes to 1 hr
Frequency	Often daily or continuous	Rarely >1/wk
Location	Nuchal or circumferential	Temporal
Character	Aching, pressure, bandlike	Pounding
Laterality	Usually bilateral	Always unilateral
Aura	Never present	May be present
Nausea and vomiting	Rare	Common
Duration	Often days	Usually <24 hr

Diseases of the cervical spine and surrounding soft tissues may also mimic tension-type headache. Arnold-Chiari malformations may manifest clinically as tension-type headache, but these malformations can easily be identified on images of the posterior fossa and cervical spine (Fig. 3.4). Occasionally, frontal sinusitis is confused with tension-type headache, although individuals with acute frontal sinusitis appear systemically ill. Temporal arteritis, chronic subdural hematoma, and other intracranial disease such as tumor may be incorrectly diagnosed as tension-type headache.

TREATMENT

Abortive therapy

In determining the best treatment, the physician must consider the frequency and severity of the headaches, their effect on the patient's lifestyle, the results of any previous therapy, and any prior drug misuse or abuse. If the patient suffers an attack of tension-type headache only once every 1 or 2 months, the condition can often be managed by teaching the patient to reduce or avoid stress. Analgesics or nonsteroidal antiinflammatory drugs (NSAIDs) can provide symptomatic relief during acute attacks. Combination analgesic drugs used concomitantly with barbiturates or opioid analgesics have no place in the treatment of patients with headache. The risk of abuse and dependence more than outweighs any theoretic benefit. The physician should also avoid an abortive treatment approach in patients with a prior history of drug misuse or abuse. Many drugs, including simple analgesics and NSAIDs, can produce serious consequences if they are abused.

Prophylactic therapy

If the headaches occur more frequently than once every 1 or 2 months or are so severe that the patient repeatedly misses work or social engagements, prophylactic therapy is indicated.

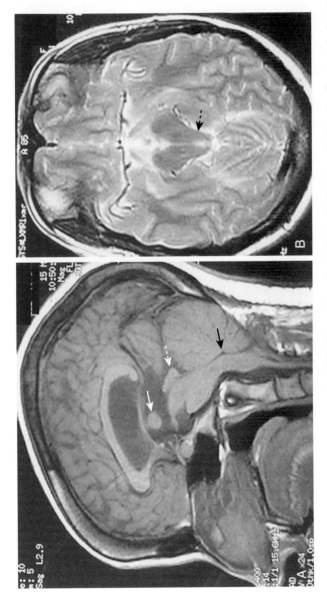

Fig. 3.4 (A) Sagittal T1-weighted magnetic resonance imaging (MRI) of an adult patient with Arnold-Chiari type II deformity. The posterior fossa is small with a widened foramen magnum. Inferior displacement of the cerebellum and medulla with elongation of the pons and fourth ventricle (black arrow) is evident. The brainstem is kinked as it passes over the back of the odontoid. An enlarged massa with intermedia (white arrow) and beaking of the tectum (broken white arrow) are visible. (B) Axial T2-weighted MRI shows the small posterior fossa with beaking of the tectum (broken black arrow). (From Waldman SD, Campbell RSD. Imaging of pain. Philadelphia: Saunders; 2011:30.)

Antidepressants

Antidepressants are generally the drugs of choice for the prophylactic treatment of tension-type headache. These drugs not only help decrease the frequency and intensity of headaches but also normalize sleep patterns and treat any underlying depression. Patients should be educated about the potential side effects of this class of drugs, including sedation, dry mouth, blurred vision, constipation, and urinary retention. Patients should also be told that relief of headache pain generally takes 3 to 4 weeks. However, normalization of sleep occurs immediately, and this may be enough to provide a noticeable improvement in headache symptoms.

Amitriptyline, started at a single bedtime dose of 25 mg, is a reasonable initial choice. The dose may be increased in 25-mg increments as side effects allow. Other drugs that can be considered if the patient does not tolerate the sedative and anticholinergic effects of amitriptyline include trazodone (75—300 mg at bedtime) or fluoxetine (20—40 mg at lunchtime). Because of the sedating nature of these drugs (with the exception of fluoxetine), they must be used with caution in older patients and in others who are at risk for falling. Care should also be exercised when using these drugs in patients who are susceptible to cardiac arrhythmias because these drugs may be arrhythmogenic. Simple analgesics or longer-acting NSAIDs may be used with antidepressant compounds to treat exacerbations of headache pain.

Biofeedback

Monitored relaxation training combined with patient education about coping strategies and stress-reduction techniques may be of value in some tension-type headache sufferers who are adequately motivated. Patient selection is of paramount importance if good results are to be achieved. If the patient is significantly depressed, it may be beneficial to treat the depression before trying biofeedback. The use of biofeedback may allow the patient to control the headaches while avoiding the side effects of medications.

Cervical epidural nerve block

Multiple studies have demonstrated the efficacy of cervical epidural nerve block with steroid in providing long-term relief of tension-type headaches in patients for whom all other treatment modalities have failed (Fig. 3.5). This treatment can also be used while waiting for antidepressant compounds to become effective. Cervical epidural nerve block can be performed on a daily to weekly basis depending on clinical symptoms.

COMPLICATIONS AND PITFALLS

A few patients with tension-type headache have major depression or uncontrolled anxiety states in addition to a chemical dependence on opioid

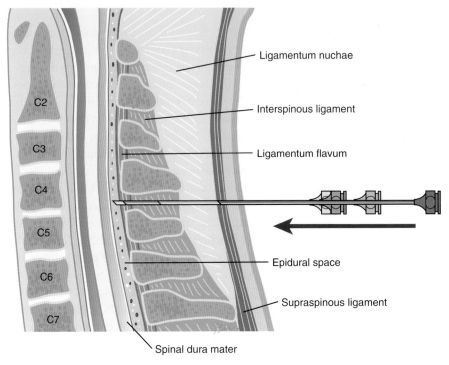

Fig. 3.5 Cervical epidural block can be useful in the palliation of tension-type headaches that are resistant to more conservative treatment modalities. (From Waldman S. *Atlas of Interventional Pain Management.* ed. 5. Philadelphia: Elsevier; 2021 [Fig. 45.5].)

analgesics, barbiturates, minor tranquilizers, or alcohol. Attempts to treat these patients in the outpatient setting are disappointing and frustrating. Inpatient treatment in a specialized headache unit or psychiatric setting results in more rapid amelioration of the underlying and coexisting problems and allows the concurrent treatment of headache. Monoamine oxidase inhibitors can often reduce the frequency and severity of tension-type headache in this subset of patients. Phenelzine, at a dosage of 15 mg three times a day, is usually effective. After 2 to 3 weeks, the dosage is tapered to an appropriate maintenance dose of 5 to 10 mg three times a day. Monoamine oxidase inhibitors can produce life-threatening hypertensive crises if special diets are not followed or if these drugs are combined with some commonly used prescription or over-the-counter medications. Therefore their use should be limited to highly reliable and com-pliant patients. Physicians prescribing this potentially dangerous group of drugs should be well versed in how to use them safely. A failure to recognize red flags can put the patient at significant risk for delayed diagnosis and harm (see Table 2.3).

HIGH-YIELD TAKEAWAYS

- The patient is afebrile, making an acute infectious etiology unlikely.
- The patient's headaches are bilateral, making a diagnosis of migraine or cluster headache unlikely.
- The character of the patient's headache pain is aching, with bandlike tightness.
- The patient does not experience other neurologic symptoms such as weakness or speech disturbance associated with her headaches.
- The patient does not have significant photophobia, nausea, or vomiting associated with her headaches.
- The patient is not experiencing significant disability associated with her headaches.
- The patient's MRI is negative.
- There are no red flags.

Suggested Readings

Burch R. Migraine and tension-type headache: diagnosis and treatment. *Med Clin North Am.* 2019;103(2):215–233.

Cuttler C, Spradlin A, Cleveland MJ, et al. Short- and long-term effects of cannabis on headache and migraine. *J Pain.* 2020;21(5–6):722–730.

Finkel AG. Botulinum toxin and the treatment of headache: a clinical review. *Toxicon.* 2015;107(Pt A):114–119.

Jay GW, Barkin RL. Primary headache disorders—part 2: tension-type headache and medication overuse headache. *Dis Month.* 2017;63(12):342–367.

Moore AR, Derry S, Wiffen PJ, et al. Evidence for efficacy of acute treatment of episodic tension-type headache: methodological critique of randomised trials for oral treatments. *Pain.* 2014;155(11):2220–2228.

Waldman SD. Cervical epidural block: translaminar approach. In: *Atlas of Interventional Pain Management.* ed. 5. Philadelphia: Elsevier; 2021:206–215.

Waldman SD. Targeted headache history. *Med Clin North Am.* 2013;97(2):185–195.

Waldman SD. Tension-type headache. In: *Atlas of Common Pain Syndromes.* ed. 4. Philadelphia: Elsevier; 2019:10–13.

Gene Fiback

A 57-Year-Old Accountant With Severe Episodic Unilateral Retro-orbital Headaches With Associated Neurologic Symptoms

- Learn the common types of headache.
- Understand the difference between primary and secondary headaches.
- Develop an understanding of clinical presentation of specific headache types.
- Develop an understanding of the treatment of specific headache types.
- Develop an understanding of the differential diagnosis of headache.
- Understand the gender predilection of specific headache types.
- Learn how to identify factors that cause concern.

Gene Fiback

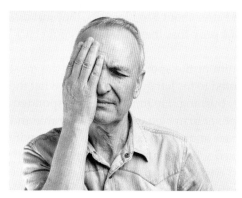

Gene Fiback is a 57-year-old accountant with the chief complaint of, "It feels like someone is jamming a red-hot poker into my eye." He explained, "Doctor, I am afraid to go to sleep at night because every night, about 90 minutes after I go to sleep, bam, the headache hits. I am sound asleep and, bam, the headache wakes me up. The pain is really bad, like nothing you can imagine. I have to get up, and I just pace. Sometimes I feel like banging my head against the wall to make the pain stop. It's really bad, unimaginably bad, like the devil is jamming a red-hot poker into my eye. It also hurts in my temple. It goes on for about an hour and then it stops. It takes me another hour to get calmed down, and I try to get some sleep. Doctor, every spring they come like clockwork and after a couple of months, they go away. And then, bam, the fall comes, and they are back again. This has been going on for the last 12 to 15 years, and I don't know how much longer I can take it. I am just so worn down."

I asked Gene if he had any symptoms other than the pain and he nodded and said that when the pain hits, the eye on his affected side waters profusely and his nose runs like crazy. "Doctor, some nights I can go through an entire box of Kleenex. My wife tells me that my face gets red and my eyelid droops. I am getting all the broken blood vessels on my face. I look like a drunk, but, Doctor, let me tell you, the last thing I am going to do is take a drink. Booze makes the headaches worse. I came in to see you with this round of headaches to see if there is anything new on the market that can help me. Over the past few years, it seems like the headaches are getting worse. Each year I get a little less headache-free time. Bam, every spring and fall like clockwork, then they go away. I pray they won't come back, but bam, there they are again. Something's got to give. I don't know how much longer I can go on." I reassured Gene that I would do everything I could to help him get these headaches under control.

I asked Gene if he had identified anything that triggered his headache and he said, "Booze definitely, high altitude for sure, I can't fly or go to Vail anymore, and as crazy as it may sound, Chinese food." I asked Gene if he knew whether he was going to get a headache before the headache actually started, and he said not really. "I am just fine when I go to bed, and bam, I get woken up from a sound sleep and I am really in trouble. The pain is just the worst."

I asked Gene what made it better, and he said, "Really nothing. I've tried all of the usual over-the-counter medications and they do absolutely nothing. The headaches come on without warning, and after about 8 to 12 weeks, they just disappear. Just like that, they are gone and I pray that they will never come back. But it's spring and here they are again."

I asked Gene to use one finger to point at the spot where it hurt the most when the headache came on and he pointed to his left eye. I asked him what the pain was like: an ache, sharp, stabbing, burning. He immediately responded, "It's like I said, bam, a burning red-hot poker in my left eye. It's unbearable and there is nothing I can do about it. I just pace and wait it out. It's driving my wife crazy. Hell, it's driving me crazy." I asked whether the headache was on both sides or just one side, and he answered emphatically, "One side. Always the one side." I asked Gene from the time that he knew he was going to get the headache until the time it was at its worst, was it a period of seconds, minutes, or hours. He said that it was usually at about 50% when it woke him up and within a minute or two, it was going full bore and he was up and out of bed, pacing back and forth, until the headache subsided. It went away "over 10 or 15 minutes." I said to Gene that several times he mentioned that the headaches were really wearing him down, so I asked if he had ever considered suicide. He said, "Yes, Doctor, but not that often. Just every time I have a headache." But he went on to say," Don't worry, Doc. I know you will get me better." I told him I would certainly try.

I asked Gene if I could examine him and he said, "Sure, but there is not much to see. I just hope you have a trick up your sleeve. You just have to get rid of these headaches. I'm just about played out." On physical examination, Gene was afebrile. His respirations were 16, and his pulse was 78 and regular. His blood pressure was 126/80. There were no cranial abnormalities. His head, eyes, ears, nose, throat (HEENT) examination was completely normal, as was his fundoscopic examination. Specifically, there was no anisocoria. His temporal arteries were normal bilaterally. I noted multiple telangiectasias on Gene's nose and cheeks, and his skin over the malar regions had a peau d'orange appearance. Deeply furrowed glabellar skin was also noted. His neck examination was normal, and no myofascial trigger points were identified. His cardiopulmonary examination was normal, as was his thyroid. There was no adenopathy. His abdominal examination revealed no abnormal mass or organomegaly, and there was no rebound tenderness present. There was no costovertebral angle (CVA) tenderness. There was no peripheral edema. A careful neurologic examination of the upper and lower extremities revealed there was no evidence of weakness, lack of coordination, or peripheral or entrapment neuropathy, and his deep tendon reflexes were normal. The remainder of his neurologic examination was completely normal. Gene's mental status exam was within normal limits.

Key Clinical Points—What's Important and What's Not

THE HISTORY

- Episodic headaches that began in the patient's late third decade
- Headaches of consistent chronobiologic pattern with peak headache occurrence in the spring and fall
- Headaches characterized by headache-free periods
- Headache consistently occurs approximately 90 minutes after the patient goes to sleep
- Headache pain is severe
- Headache is unilateral
- Headache is retro-orbital with a deep burning, stabbing quality
- Headaches are associated with profuse lacrimation and rhinorrhea on the affected side
- No prodrome or aura
- No fever or chills
- Patient denies significant nausea and vomiting associated with the headache
- Headaches associated with suicidal ideation

THE PHYSICAL EXAMINATION

- Patient is afebrile
- Normal fundoscopic exam
- Examination of the cranium is normal
- Neurologic exam is normal
- Telangiectasias over patient's nose and cheeks
- Peau d'orange appearance of skin over malar areas
- Deeply furrowed glabellar skin

OTHER FINDINGS OF NOTE

- Normal cardiovascular examination
- Normal pulmonary examination
- Normal abdominal examination
- No peripheral edema
- Normal upper and lower extremity neurologic examination, motor and sensory examination

 ## What Tests Would You Like to Order?

The following test was ordered:
- Magnetic resonance imaging (MRI) of the brain

TEST RESULTS

The MRI of the brain was normal.

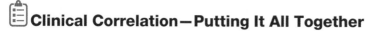

Clinical Correlation—Putting It All Together

What is the diagnosis?
  Cluster headache

The Science Behind the Diagnosis

CLINICAL SYNDROME

Cluster headache derives its name from the headache pattern—that is, head-aches occur in clusters, followed by headache-free remission periods. Cluster headache is a primary headache that is included in the group of headaches known as the trigeminal autonomic cephalgias. Unlike other common headache disorders that affect primarily female patients, cluster headache is much more common in male patients, with a male-to-female ratio of 5:1. Much less common than tension-type headache or migraine headache, cluster headache is thought to affect approximately 0.5% of the male population. Cluster headache is most often confused with migraine by clinicians who are unfamiliar with the syn-drome; however, a targeted headache history allows the clinician to distinguish between these two distinct headache types easily (Table 4.1).

The onset of cluster headache occurs in the late third or early fourth decade of life, in contradistinction from migraine, which almost always manifests by the early second decade. Unlike migraine, cluster headache does not appear to run in families, and cluster headache sufferers do not experience auras. Attacks gen-erally occur approximately 90 minutes after the patient falls asleep. This associa-tion with sleep is reportedly maintained when a shift worker changes from

TABLE 4.1 ■ Comparison of Cluster Headache and Migraine Headache

	Cluster Headache	Migraine Headache
Gender	Male 5:1	Female 2:1
Age of onset	Late 30s to early 40s	Menarche to early 20s
Family history	No	Yes
Aura	Never	May be present (20% of the time)
Chronobiologic pattern	Yes	No
Onset-to-peak interval	Seconds to minutes	Minutes to 1 hr
Frequency	2 or 3/day	Rarely >1/wk
Duration	45 min	Usually <24 hr

nighttime to daytime hours of sleep. Cluster headache also appears to follow a distinct chronobiologic pattern that coincides with seasonal changes in the length of the day. This pattern results in an increased frequency of cluster headache in the spring and fall.

During a cluster period, attacks occur two or three times a day and last for 45 minutes to 1 hour. Cluster periods usually last for 8 to 12 weeks, interrupted by remission periods of less than 2 years. In rare patients, the remission periods become shorter and shorter, and the frequency may increase up to 10-fold. This situation is termed *chronic cluster headache* and differs from the more common episodic cluster headache described earlier.

SIGNS AND SYMPTOMS

Cluster headache is characterized as a unilateral headache that is retro-orbital and temporal in location. The pain has a deep burning or boring quality. Physical findings during an attack of cluster headache may include Horner syndrome, consisting of ptosis, abnormal pupil constriction, facial flushing, and conjunctival injection (Fig. 4.1). Additionally, profuse lacrimation and rhinorrhea are often present. The ocular changes may become permanent with repeated attacks. Peau d'orange skin over the malar region, deeply furrowed glabellar folds, and telangiectasia may be observed. The exact etiology of cluster headache remains elusive, but it is thought to be related to activation of the trigemino-vascular and trigeminal autonomic reflex.

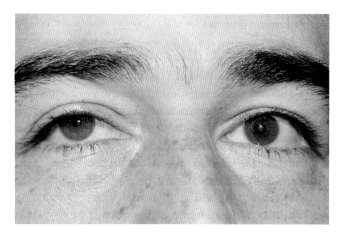

Fig. 4.1 Horner syndrome eye findings. Classic clinical eye findings are demonstrated in this patient with a right Horner syndrome (ptosis of the upper eyelid, elevation of the lower eyelid, and miosis). (From Reede DL, Garcon E, Smoker WR, et al. Horner's syndrome: clinical and radiographic evaluation. *Neuroimaging Clin N Am.* 2008; 18(2):369–385.)

Attacks of cluster headache may be provoked by small amounts of alcohol, nitrates, histamines, and other vasoactive substances, as well as occasionally by high altitude. When the attack is in progress, the patient may be unable to lie still and may pace or rock back and forth in a chair. This behavior contrasts with that characterizing other headache syndromes, during which patients seek relief by lying down in a dark, quiet room. The pain of cluster headache is said to be among the worst pain a human being can suffer. Because of the severity of the pain, the clinician must watch closely for medication overuse or misuse. Suicide has been associated with prolonged, unrelieved attacks of cluster headache.

TESTING

No specific test exists for cluster headache. Testing is aimed primarily at identifying an occult pathologic process or other diseases that may mimic cluster headache (see "Differential Diagnosis") (Fig. 4.2). All patients with a recent onset of headache thought to be a cluster headache should undergo MRI of the brain. If neurologic dysfunction accompanies the patient's headache symptoms, MRI should be performed with and without gadolinium contrast medium (Fig. 4.3); magnetic resonance angiography and computed tomography (CT) angiography should be considered as well. MRI should also be performed in patients with previously stable cluster headache who experience an inexplicable change in symptoms. Screening laboratory tests, including an erythrocyte sedimentation rate, complete blood count, and automated blood chemistry, should be performed if the diagnosis of cluster headache is in question. Ophthalmologic evaluation, including measurement of intraocular pressures, is indicated in patients who experience significant ocular symptoms.

DIFFERENTIAL DIAGNOSIS

Cluster headache is usually diagnosed on clinical grounds by obtaining a targeted headache history. Migraine headache is often confused with cluster headache, and this misdiagnosis can lead to illogic treatment plans because the management of these two headache syndromes is quite different. Table 4.1 distinguishes cluster headache from migraine headache and should help clarify the diagnosis.

Diseases of the eyes, ears, nose, and sinuses may also mimic cluster headache. The targeted history and physical examination, combined with appropriate testing, should help an astute clinician identify and properly treat any underlying diseases of these organ systems. The following conditions may all mimic cluster headache and must be considered in patients with headache: glaucoma, temporal arteritis, sinusitis (see Fig. 4.2), intracranial disease (including aneurysm, chronic subdural hematoma, tumor, brain abscess, hydrocephalus, and pseudotumor cerebri), and inflammatory conditions (including sarcoidosis).

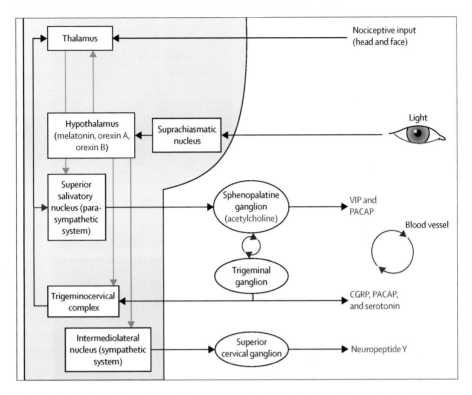

Fig. 4.2 Anatomic and neurotransmitter components of cluster headache pathophysiology. The superior salivatory nucleus (parasympathetic system), trigeminocervical complex, and intermediolateral nucleus (sympathetic system) are under the control of the hypothalamus, which communicates with the suprachiasmatic nucleus. A strong trigeminal nociceptive input from the head and face generates a signal that is transmitted to the thalamus. This signal is generated in the periphery, but also centrally, which results in parasympathetic outflow. This parasympathetic reaction (lacrimation, conjunctival injection) could be facilitated by the sympathetic deficit (miosis, ptosis) that is inherent to cluster attacks. Neurotransmitters known to be involved in cluster headache are shown (e.g., acetylcholine, serotonin, neuropeptide Y). Words in red are neurotransmitters, and words in black are anatomic structures. Black arrows are connections between peripheral and central nervous systems. Blue arrows indicate central brainstem connections. Red arrows indicate connected structures within the brainstem. Red arrows in a circle illustrate the trigeminal autonomic reflex. CGRP, Calcitonin gene–related peptide; PACAP, pituitary adenylate cyclase-activating peptide; VIP, vasoactive intestinal peptide. (Reprinted with permission from Elsevier (From Hoffmann J, May A. Diagnosis, pathophysiology, and management of cluster headache. *Lancet Neurol.* 2018;17(1):7583 [Fig. 2]. ISSN 1474-4422).)

TREATMENT

Whereas most patients with migraine headache experience improvement with beta-blocker therapy, patients suffering from cluster headache usually require more individualized therapy. Initial treatment is commonly prednisone combined with daily sphenopalatine ganglion blocks with local anesthetic (Fig. 4.4).

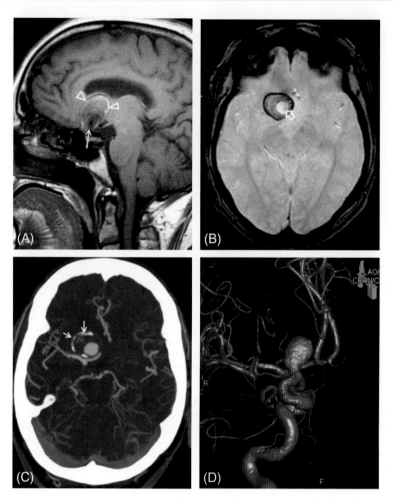

Fig. 4.3 Magnetic resonance imaging (MRI) and computed tomography angiograph (CTA) of an intracranial aneurysm. Axial GRE T2 (A), sagittal precontrast T1 MRI (B), axial CTA MIP (C), and 3DRA frontal projection (D) show a partially thrombosed giant aneurysm of the right carotid terminus. Note eccentric lumen *(hollow arrow)* with concentric layers of mural thrombus on MRI and peripheral calcification on CTA *(arrows)*. The hyperintense T1 rind on the periphery represents the most recent thrombus *(arrowheads in B)*. (From Ringer A. *Intracranial Aneurysms*. London: Academic Press; 2018 [Fig. 5-5]. 9780128117408.)

A reasonable starting dose of prednisone is 80 mg given in divided doses and tapered by 10 mg/dose per day. If headaches are not rapidly brought under control, inhalation of 100% oxygen through a close-fitting mask is added. Octreotide, a synthetic form of somatostatin, may also be useful in aborting acute attacks of cluster headache. Clinical trials suggest that the new monoclonal antibodies against calcitonin gene—related peptide drugs, fremanezumab and

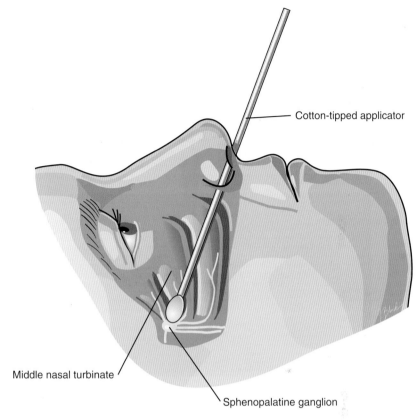

Fig. 4.4   Sphenopalatine ganglion block is a useful treatment in the management of cluster headache. (From Waldman SD. *Atlas of interventional pain management*. 4th ed. Philadelphia: Elsevier; 2015.)

galcanezumab, may be useful in the treatment of cluster headache. Implantation of neurostimulators also shows promise in selected cases (Fig. 4.5).

COMPLICATIONS AND PITFALLS

The major risk in patients suffering from uncontrolled cluster headache is that they may become despondent owing to the unremitting, severe pain and commit suicide. Therefore, if the clinician has difficulty controlling the patient's pain, hospitalization should be considered. Cluster headache represents one of the most painful conditions encountered in clinical practice and must be viewed as a true pain emergency. In general, cluster headache is more difficult to treat than migraine headache and requires more individualized therapy. Given the severity of the pain associated with cluster headache, multiple modalities should be used early in the course of an episode of cluster headache. The clinician should

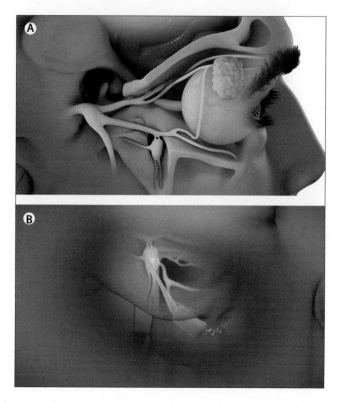

Fig. 4.5   (A) Anatomy relevant to implantation of the sphenopalatine ganglion stimulation system. (B) Proper positioning for sphenopalatine ganglion stimulation electrode. (Reprinted with permission from Elsevier (From Goadsby PJ, Sahai Srivastava S, Kezirian EJ, et al. Safety and efficacy of sphenopalatine ganglion stimulation for chronic cluster headache: a double-blind, randomised controlled trial. *Lancet Neurol.* 2019;18(12):1081–1090 Fig. 2).)

beware of patients presenting with a classic history of cluster headache who request opioid analgesics.

HIGH-YIELD TAKEAWAYS

- The patient is afebrile, making an acute infectious etiology unlikely.
- The patient is a male.
- The patient's headaches are unilateral, making a diagnosis of tension-type headache unlikely.
- The character of the patient's headache pain is severe burning and stabbing retro-orbital pain.

(Continued)

- The patient's headaches have a classic chronobiologic pattern, occuring in spring and fall.
- The patient's headaches occur approximately 90 minutes after the patient falls asleep.
- The patient's headaches have a rapid onset to peak of minutes.
- The patient's headaches are associated with the onset of Horner syndrome.
- The patient's headaches are associated with profuse lacrimation and rhinorrhea.
- The patient does not have significant photophobia and nausea and vomiting associated with his headaches, as is commonly seen in migraine headache.
- The patient's MRI is negative.
- The patient admits to suicide ideation because of the severity and frequency of headache.

Suggested Readings

Belvis R, Rodríguez R, Guasch M, et al. Efficacy and safety of surgical treatment of cluster headache. *Medicina Clínica* (English Ed.). 2020;154(3):75−79.

Forde G, Duarte RA, Rosen N. Managing chronic headache disorders. *Med Clin North Am.* 2016;100(1):117−141.

Goadsby PJ, Sahai-Srivastava S, Kezirian EJ, et al. Safety and efficacy of sphenopalatine ganglion stimulation for chronic cluster headache: a double-blind, randomised controlled trial. *Lancet Neurol.* 2019;18(1):1081−1090.

Hoffmann J, May A. Diagnosis, pathophysiology, and management of cluster headache. *Lancet Neurol.* 2018;17(1):75−83.

Waldman SD. Cluster headache. In: *Atlas of Common Pain Syndromes.* ed. 4. Philadelphia: Elsevier; 2019:14−17.

Waldman SD. Sphenopalatine ganglion block—transnasal approach. In: *Atlas of Interventional Pain Management.* ed. 5. Philadelphia: Elsevier; 2021:13−16.

Waldman SD. Targeted headache history. *Med Clin North Am.* 2013;97(2):185−195.

Jeff Baker

A 24-Year-Old Medical Student With Severe Episodic Headache Associated With Sexual Activity

- Learn the common types of headache.
- Understand the difference between primary and secondary headaches.
- Develop an understanding of clinical presentation of specific headache types.
- Develop an understanding of the treatment of specific headache types.
- Develop an understanding of the differential diagnosis of primary headaches.
- Understand the gender predilection of specific headache types.
- Learn how to identify factors that cause concern.

Jeff Baker

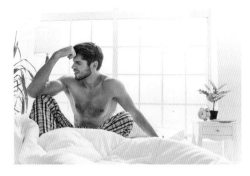

Jeff Baker is a 24-year-old medical student with the chief complaint of headache associated with sexual activity. Jeff shook hands with me and said, "Doctor, I have one for you. It's kind of embarrassing to talk about, but my partner is really worried about me and wanted me to see if you could help." I reassured Jeff that I would certainly try and that whatever it was he was in a judgment-free zone, so there was nothing to be embarrassed about. I also reassured him that anything we discussed would be held in the strictest confidence. He seemed to relax a bit, so I said, "Jeff, tell me what's going on and together we will get it sorted out."

"Well, whenever I have sex, when I start to really get excited, I start to get this dull pain in my occipital area and neck, and if I keep going it spreads and gets really intense—not the sex, the headache. The headache is not helping the sex at all; it's a real party pooper, if you know what I mean." "Do you mean inability to get an erection?" I asked, and he said, "Not so much that, but I am starting to be afraid to have sex. I don't want to have a stroke or anything. Like I said, my partner is really worried about me, but is getting frustrated about the sex thing." I nodded and said that I understood.

I asked Jeff if he had any symptoms associated with the headache and he shook his head. "Doctor, there is no aura, if that is what you are asking. No photophobia, sonophobia, or osmophobia like migraine. My diagnosis is this is not migraine." I smiled and said that I was glad he didn't sleep through his neurology lectures. He laughed and seemed more relaxed. I asked if the headache occurred with all sexual activity, masturbation, oral sex, or just with sexual intercourse and he said it happened with all types of sexual activity. "The more excited I get, the worse the headache gets." I asked about any other constitutional symptoms or neurologic symptoms, and Jeff said no. He also denied the use of erectile dysfunction drugs or the use of illicit drugs during sexual activity, including cocaine and amyl nitrate poppers.

I asked Jeff what made his headache better, and he said, "Really nothing, other than avoiding sex. No sex, no headache. I've tried all the usual over-the-counter medications and they do absolutely nothing—not before I have sex or when the headache starts."

I asked Jeff to use one finger to point at the spot where it hurt the most when the headache came on, and he pointed to the occipital region. "Both sides, Doc, and then down into the neck and up to the vertex of the scalp." I asked Jeff what the pain was like and he said it started as an ache and increased in intensity as he got more sexually excited. I asked if it was associated with orgasm and he said no, it was at its worst just before orgasm and then gradually subsided after orgasm. "Like I said, this is not helping my sex life and I feel bad for my partner having to deal with this."

I said, "Let's look you over."

I asked Jeff if I could examine him and he said, "Sure, but there is not much to see." On physical examination, Jeff was afebrile. His respirations were 16 and his pulse was 70 and regular. His blood pressure was 118/70. There were no cranial abnormalities. His head, eyes, ears, nose, throat (HEENT) examination was completely normal, as was his fundoscopic examination. Temporal arteries were normal bilaterally. His neck examination was normal, and no myofascial trigger points were identified. His cardiopulmonary examination was normal, as was his thyroid. There was no adenopathy. His abdominal examination revealed no abnormal mass or organomegaly, and there was no rebound tenderness present. There was no costovertebral angle (CVA) tenderness. There was no peripheral edema. A careful neurologic examination of the upper and lower extremities revealed no evidence of weakness, lack of coordination, or peripheral or entrapment neuropathy, and his deep tendon reflexes were normal. The remainder of his neurologic examination was completely normal.

I reassured Jeff that I didn't find anything on physical examination that was cause for concern. "So, Jeff, I have a pretty good idea what is going on and what to do about it, but I'm curious. What is your diagnosis?" Jeff said, "Either sexual headache or I've got a leaky aneurysm." I said, "Jeff, I think we should go with the first one!"

Key Clinical Points—What's Important and What's Not

THE HISTORY

- Episodic headache associated with all sexual activity
- Headache that worsens during sexual excitement, but orgasm does not affect intensity
- No prodrome or aura
- Severe headache pain
- Bilateral headache
- Headache that begins as a suboccipital ache but progresses during increasing sexual excitement to involve the neck
- Headache not associated with neurologic signs or symptoms
- Patient denies fever, chills, or other constitutional symptoms
- Patient denies significant nausea and vomiting associated with headache

THE PHYSICAL EXAMINATION

- Patient is afebrile
- Normal fundoscopic exam
- Examination of the cranium is normal
- Neurologic exam is normal

OTHER FINDINGS OF NOTE

- Normal cardiovascular examination
- Normal pulmonary examination
- Normal abdominal examination
- No peripheral edema

 What Tests Would You Like to Order?

The following test was ordered:
- Magnetic resonance imaging (MRI) of the brain

TEST RESULTS

The MRI of the brain was normal.

 Clinical Correlation—Putting It All Together

What is the diagnosis?
Sexual headache

The Science Behind the Diagnosis

CLINICAL SYNDROME

Sexual headache is a term used to describe a group of headaches associated with sexual activity. Sexual headache is also known as primary headache associated with sexual activity, benign vascular sexual headache, coital cephalalgia, coital headache, intercourse headache, (pre)orgasmic cephalalgia, and (pre)orgasmic headache (Fig. 5.1). Clinicians have identified the following three general types of headache associated with sexual activity: (1) explosive type, (2) dull type, and (3) postural type, with each type having a preorgasmic and an orgasmic variant. In general, sexual headache includes a benign group of disorders, but a rare patient may have acute subarachnoid hemorrhage during sexual activity, which may be erroneously diagnosed as the benign

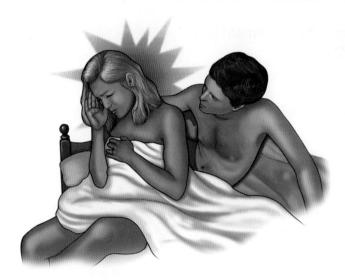

Fig. 5.1   Sexual headache is a term used to describe a group of episodic headaches that are associated with sexual activity. (From Waldman S. *Atlas of Uncommon Pain Syndromes*. ed. 4. Philadelphia: Elsevier; 2020 [Fig. 6.1]. 9780323640770.)

explosive type of sexual headache (Fig. 5.2). There is a slight gender predilection for males suffering sexual headache, and the occurrence of all types of sexual headache may be episodic rather than chronic. Rarely, more than one type of sexual headache occurs in the same patient. Sexual headaches have been associated with the use of cannabis, pseudoephedrine, oral contraceptives, and amiodarone.

SIGNS AND SYMPTOMS

Patients with sexual headache present differently depending on the type of sexual headache experienced (Table 5.1). Each clinical presentation is discussed subsequently.

Explosive type of sexual headache

The explosive type of sexual headache is the most common type encountered in clinical practice. The patient usually fears a stroke has occurred. The patient may be less forthcoming about the circumstances surrounding the onset of headache, and tactful questioning may be required to ascertain the actual clinical history. The explosive type of sexual headache occurs suddenly, with an almost instantaneous onset to peak just before or during orgasm. The intensity of the explosive type of sexual headache is severe and has been likened to the pain of acute subarachnoid hemorrhage. The location of pain is usually occipital, but some

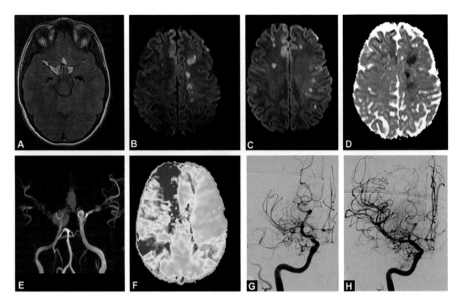

Fig. 5.2 A 29-year-old woman presenting with a subarachnoid hemorrhage, initially Fisher grade 3 due to rupture of the anterior communicating artery treated endovascularly *(not shown)*. On D10, she developed a left hemiplegia. Urgent cerebral magnetic resonance imaging reveals: Appearance of subarachnoid hemorrhage, hyperintense of FLAIR imaging in the motor cortex sulci (A). Development of bilateral junctional hyperintense b1000 punctiform ischemic lesions (B, C); restriction on ADC mapping (D). Pronounced spasm of the trunks of the carotid arteries and middle and anterior cerebral arteries seen on time of flight imaging of the circle of Willis (E) with large extensive increase in the mean transit time mostly affecting the middle and right anterior cerebral artery territories and the left posterior superficial middle cerebral artery (F). Confirmation of severe spasm of the carotid and middle and right anterior cerebral artery trunks on arteriography performed immediately afterwards (G) and a large improvement in cerebral parenchymography after intraarterial injection of milrinone (H). (From Danière F, Gascou G, Menjot de Champfleur N, et al. Complications and followup of subarachnoid hemorrhages. *Diagn Interv Imaging.* 2015;96[7-8]:677—686 [Fig. 4]. ISSN 2211-5684, https://doi.org/10.1016/j.diii.2015.05.006. http://www.sciencedirect.com/science/article/pii/S2211568415001990)

TABLE 5.1 ■ Types of Sexual Headache

Explosive type
    Preorgasmic
    Orgasmic
Dull type
    Preorgasmic
    Orgasmic
Postural type
    Preorgasmic
    Orgasmic

patients volunteer that the pain felt "like the top of my head was going to blow off." The pain is usually bilateral, but isolated cases of unilateral explosive sexual headache have been reported. The pain usually remains intense for 10 to 15 minutes and then gradually abates. Some patients note some residual headache pain for 2 days.

Dull type of sexual headache

The dull type of sexual headache begins during the early portion of sexual activity. This headache type has an aching character and begins in the occipital region. The headache becomes holocranial as sexual activity progresses toward orgasm. It may peak at orgasm, but in contrast to the explosive type of sexual headache, the dull type disappears rapidly after orgasm. Ceasing sexual activity usually aborts the dull type of sexual headache. Some headache specialists think the dull type of sexual headache is simply a milder version of the explosive type of sexual headache.

Postural type of sexual headache

The postural type of sexual headache is similar to the explosive type in that it occurs just before or during orgasm. Its rapid onset to peak and severe intensity also are similar to that of the explosive type. It differs from the explosive type of headache in that the headache symptoms recur when the patient stands up, in a manner analogous to postdural puncture headache. The postural component of this type of sexual headache is thought to be due to minute tears in the dura that may occur during intense sexual activity.

TESTING

Magnetic resonance imaging of the brain provides the best information regarding the cranial vault and its contents. MRI is highly accurate and helps identify abnormalities that may put the patient at risk for neurologic disasters secondary to intracranial and brainstem pathologic conditions, including tumors, demyelinating disease, and hemorrhage. More important, MRI helps identify bleeding associated with leaking intracranial aneurysms. Magnetic resonance angiography (MRA) may be useful in helping identify aneurysms responsible for the patient's neurologic symptoms. In patients who cannot undergo MRI, such as patients with pacemakers, computed tomography (CT) is a reasonable second choice. Even if blood is not present on MRI or CT, if intracranial hemorrhage is suspected, then lumbar puncture should be performed. Screening laboratory tests consisting of complete blood cell count, erythrocyte sedimentation rate, and automated blood chemistry testing should be performed if the diagnosis of sexual headache is in question. Intraocular pressure should be measured if glaucoma is suspected.

DIFFERENTIAL DIAGNOSIS

Sexual headache is a clinical diagnosis supported by a combination of clinical history, normal physical examination, radiography, MRI, and MRA. Pain syndromes that may mimic sexual headache include trigeminal neuralgia involving the first division of the trigeminal nerve, demyelinating disease, cluster headache, migraine, and chronic paroxysmal hemicrania. Trigeminal neuralgia involving the first division of the trigeminal nerve is uncommon and is characterized by trigger areas and ticlike movements. Demyelinating disease is generally associated with other neurologic findings, including optic neuritis and other motor and sensory abnormalities. The pain of chronic paroxysmal hemicrania and cluster headache is associated with redness and watering of the ipsilateral eye, nasal congestion, and rhinorrhea during the headache. These findings are absent in all types of sexual headache. Migraine headache may or may not be associated with nonpainful neurologic findings known as aura, but the patient almost always reports some systemic symptoms, such as nausea or photophobia, not typically associated with sexual headache. Sexual headache should be distinguished from pornography headache, which is a rare type of primary headache characterized by the onset of preorgasmic headache that is triggered by the viewing of pornography containing specific erotic content associated rather than being triggered by sexual activity. Interestingly, the intensity of pornography headache appears to be directly related to the specific erotic content being viewed. Pornography headache is thought to be a result of visuoneural uncoupling resulting in sexual arousal–mediated vascular dysregulation.

TREATMENT

It is generally thought that avoiding the inciting activity for a few weeks decreases the propensity to trigger sexual headaches. If this avoidance technique fails or is impractical because of patient preference, a trial of propranolol is a reasonable next step. A low dose of 20 to 40 mg as a daily dose and titrating in 20-mg increments to 200 mg as a divided daily dose until prophylaxis occurs treats most patients suffering from sexual headache. Propranolol should be used with caution in patients with asthma or cardiac failure and in patients with brittle diabetes.

If propranolol is ineffective, indomethacin may be tried. A starting dose of 25 mg daily for 2 days and titrating to 25 mg three times per day is a reasonable treatment approach. This dose may be carefully increased to 150 mg per day. Indomethacin must be used carefully, if at all, in patients with peptic ulcer disease or impaired renal function. Anecdotal reports of a positive response to cyclo-oxygenase-2 (COX-2) inhibitors in the treatment of sexual headache have been noted in the headache literature. Underlying sleep disturbance and depression are best treated with a tricyclic antidepressant compound, such as nortriptyline, which can be started at a single bedtime dose of 25 mg.

COMPLICATIONS AND PITFALLS

Failure to diagnose sexual headache correctly may put the patient at risk of intra-cranial pathology or demyelinating disease (which may mimic the clinical presentation of sexual headache) being overlooked. MRI and MRA are indicated in all patients thought to have sexual headache. Failure to diagnose glaucoma, which also may cause intermittent ocular pain, may result in permanent loss of sight.

HIGH-YIELD TAKEAWAYS

- The patient is afebrile, making an acute infectious etiology unlikely.
- The headaches are associated with sexual activity.
- The patient is male.
- The patient's headaches are bilateral, making a diagnosis of migraine or cluster headache unlikely.
- The character of the patient's headache pain is aching in nature.
- The patient's headache pain increases with increasing sexual excitement during sexual activity.
- The patient's headaches have a rapid onset to peak of minutes.
- The patient does not have significant photophobia and nausea and vomiting associated with the headaches, as is commonly seen in migraine headache.
- The patient's MRI is negative.

Suggested Readings

Chen W-H, Chen KY, Yin H-L. Pornography headache. *Clin Neurol Neurosurg*. 2018;164: 11–13.

Delasobera BE, Osborn SR, Davis JE. Thunderclap headache with orgasm: a case of bas-ilar artery dissection associated with sexual intercourse. *J Emerg Med*. 2012;43(1): e43–e47.

Evans RW. Diagnostic testing for migraine and other primary headaches. *Neurol Clin*. 2019;37(4):707–725.

González-Quintanilla V, Pascual J. Other primary headaches: an update. *Neurol Clin*. 2019;37(4):871–891.

Hu CM, Lin YJ, Fan YK, et al. Isolated thunderclap headache during sex: orgasmic headache or reversible cerebral vasoconstriction syndrome? *J Clin Neurosci*. 2010;17 (10):1349–1351.

Jolobe OMP. The differential diagnosis includes reversible cerebral vasoconstrictor syn-drome. *Am J Emerg Med*. 2010;28(5):637.

Kim HJ, Seo SY. Recurrent emotion-triggered headache following primary headache associated with sexual activity. *J Neurol Sci.* 2008;273(1-2):142–143.

Tuğba T, Serap Ü, Esra O, et al. Features of stabbing, cough, exertional and sexual headaches in a Turkish population of headache patients. *J Clin Neurosci.* 2008;15 (7):774–777.

Waldman SD. Sexual headache. In: *Atlas of Uncommon Pain Syndromes.* ed. 4. Philadelphia: Elsevier; 2021:17–19.

Waldman SD. Targeted headache history. *Med Clin North Am.* 2013;97(2):185–195.

Brooke Johnson

A 30-Year-Old Teacher With Frequent Headaches Involving the Head and Neck

- Learn the common types of headache.
- Understand the difference between primary and secondary headaches.
- Develop an understanding of clinical presentation of specific headache types.
- Develop an understanding of the treatment of specific headache types.
- Develop an understanding of the differential diagnosis of headache.
- Develop an understanding of the potential risks of abortive therapy in the treatment of chronic headache.
- Learn how to identify factors that cause concern.

Brooke Johnson

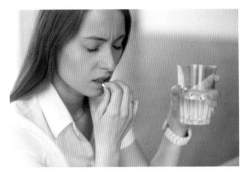

Brooke Johnson is a 30-year-old teacher with the chief complaint of, "My headache medications quit working." Brooke went on to say that she couldn't remember the last time that she didn't have a headache. "Doctor, anymore, I have a headache 24/7. It doesn't matter how much medication I take, my headaches keep coming back. The headaches make it impossible to concentrate. I'm cranky with everyone, and everyone is driving me crazy. I'm anxious all of the time."

I asked Brooke how long she's had headaches and she said, "I've had headaches about as long as I can remember." Brooke said that all of the headache medication she was taking was "eating a hole in my stomach. I take my Fiorinal and Advil, and my headache gets better for a few minutes and then it is back as bad as ever. I take some more, the headache gets better for a few minutes and then it comes right back." She denied any fever, chills, or neurologic symptoms associated with her headaches.

I asked Brooke to use one finger to point at the spot where it hurt the most, and she pointed to both her temples and then started rubbing her neck. I asked her what the pain was like: an ache, sharp, stabbing, burning? She immediately said, "My entire head just hurts! It just hurts. No throbbing, no stabbing, it just hurts. And my meds don't work. No matter how many I take! I am really up the creek here. Oh, and don't let me forget that I need you to refill my Fiorinal." I asked whether the headache was on both sides or just one side, and she said it was the entire head. I asked Brooke from the time that she knew that she was going to get the headache until the time it was at its worst, was it a period of seconds, minutes, or hours. She said, "Like I told you, I get the headache, I take my headache meds, it gets better for a bit, and then the same headache starts to come back. I take more meds, the headache gets better for a bit, it comes back, and then I take more meds to try and get some relief. I feel like a hamster on a wheel; this is the pits." I asked Brooke how her sleep was, and she replied, "Who has time to sleep? I'm too busy getting up to take my headache pills. Oh, and before I forget, I need you to refill my Fiorinal."

On physical examination, Brooke was afebrile. Her respirations were 16 and her pulse was 78 and regular. Her blood pressure was 128/82. There were no cranial abnormalities, and her head, eyes, ears, nose, throat (HEENT) examination was completely normal, as was her fundoscopic examination. Her cervical paraspinous muscles were tender to deep palpation, but no myofascial trigger points were identified. Her cardiopulmonary examination was normal, as was her thyroid. Her abdominal examination revealed no abnormal mass or organomegaly, and there was no rebound tenderness present. There was no costovertebral angle (CVA) tenderness. There was no peripheral edema. A careful neurologic examination of the upper and lower extremities revealed no evidence of weakness, lack of coordination, or peripheral or entrapment neuropathy, and her deep tendon reflexes were normal. There were no pathologic reflexes. Brooke's mental status exam was within normal limits, but her anxiety was apparent.

Key Clinical Points—What's Important and What's Not

THE HISTORY

- Episodic headaches entire adult life
- A recent increase in the intake of headache medications and over-the-counter analgesics to treat an increase in the intensity and frequency of her previously controlled headaches
- Headaches are holocranial
- Headaches are associated with some nuchal pain
- Character of the headache pain was neither sharp nor throbbing
- No neurologic symptoms associated with headache
- Significant sleep disturbance
- Patient denies fever or chills
- Patient denies significant nausea and vomiting associated with headache

THE PHYSICAL EXAMINATION

- The patient is afebrile
- Normal fundoscopic exam
- Examination of the cranium is normal
- Neurologic exam is normal
- Some tenderness of the paraspinous muscles without myofascial trigger points
- The patient appeared anxious

OTHER FINDINGS OF NOTE

- Normal cardiovascular examination
- Normal pulmonary examination
- Normal abdominal examination
- No peripheral edema
- Normal upper and lower extremity neurologic examination, motor and sensory examination

What Tests Would You Like to Order?

The following test was ordered:
- Magnetic resonance imaging (MRI) of the brain

TEST RESULTS

The MRI of the brain was normal.

 Clinical Correlation—Putting It All Together

What is the diagnosis?
Medication overuse (analgesic rebound) headache

The Science Behind the Diagnosis
CLINICAL SYNDROME

Medication overuse headache, which is also known as analgesic rebound headache, is a problematic secondary headache syndrome that occurs in headache sufferers who overuse abortive medications to treat their symptoms. It is estimated that over 60 million people suffer from medication overuse headache. The overuse of these medications results in increasingly frequent headaches that become unresponsive to both abortive and prophylactic medications. Over a period of weeks, the patient's episodic migraine or tension-type primary headache syndrome becomes more frequent and transforms into a chronic daily headache. This daily headache becomes increasingly unresponsive to analgesics and other medications, and the patient notes an exacerbation of headache symptoms if abortive or prophylactic analgesic medications are missed or delayed (Fig. 6.1). Medication overuse headache is more common in females and in headache sufferers with comorbid depression, anxiety, and other chronic pain conditions. Metabolic syndrome and regular use of benzodiazepines may also predispose patients to medication overuse headache. Some investigators believe the frequency of headaches and the total number of medications taken on a daily basis may serve as a predictor for patients suffering from medication overuse headache and who are likely to relapse. Other investigators believe that medication overuse headache is a behavioral problem due to the commonly seen compulsive drug-seeking behavior, withdrawal symptoms, and high relapse rates. Although the exact underlying pathophysiology responsible for the evolution of medication overuse headache has not been fully elucidated, it has been postulated that dysfunction of the mesolimbic-cortical dopaminergic reward circuitry as well as the trigeminal modulating system and central sensitization may play a role. Medication overuse headache is probably underdiagnosed by

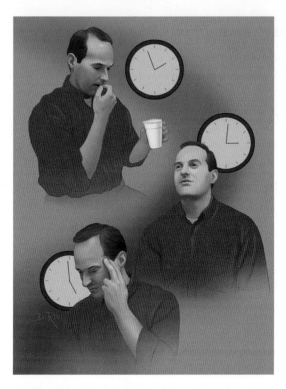

Fig. 6.1 Classic temporal relationship between the taking of abortive medications and the onset of analgesic rebound headache. (From Waldman S. *Atlas of Common Pain Syndromes*. ed. 4. Philadelphia: Elsevier; 2019 [Fig. 6-1]. 9780323547314.)

health care professionals, and its frequency is on the rise owing to the heavy advertising of over-the-counter headache medications containing caffeine.

SIGNS AND SYMPTOMS

Clinically, analgesic rebound headache manifests as a transformed migraine or tension-type headache and may assume the characteristics of both these common headache types, thus blurring their distinctive features and making diagnosis difficult. Common to all analgesic rebound headaches is the excessive use of any of the following medications: simple analgesics, such as acetaminophen; sinus medications, including simple analgesics; combinations of aspirin, caffeine, and butalbital (Fiorinal); nonsteroidal antiinflammatory drugs; opioid analgesics; ergotamines; and triptans, such as sumatriptan (Box 6.1). As with migraine and tension-type headache, the physical examination is usually within normal limits, although psychiatric comorbidities as well as compulsive drug-seeking behavior may be more prevalent in this group of headache sufferers.

BOX 6.1 ■ Drugs Implicated in Medication Overuse Headache

Simple analgesics
Nonsteroidal antiinflammatory drugs
Opioid analgesics
Sinus medications
Ergotamines
Combination headache medications that include butalbital
Triptans (e.g., sumatriptan)

TESTING

No specific test exists for analgesic rebound headache. Testing is aimed primarily at identifying an occult pathologic process or other diseases that may mimic tension-type or migraine headaches (see "Differential Diagnosis"). All patients with the recent onset of chronic daily headaches thought to be analgesic rebound headaches should undergo MRI of the brain and, if significant occipital or nuchal symptoms are present, of the cervical spine. MRI should also be performed in patients with previously stable tension-type or migraine headaches who have experienced a recent change in headache symptoms. Recent research has suggested that MRI diffusion tensor imaging may be useful in the diagnosis of patients suffering with medication overuse headache with migraine as the primary underlying headache. Screening laboratory tests consisting of a complete blood count, erythrocyte sedimentation rate, and automated blood chemistry should be performed if the diagnosis of analgesic rebound headache is in question (Fig. 6.2).

DIFFERENTIAL DIAGNOSIS

Analgesic rebound headache is usually diagnosed on clinical grounds by obtaining a targeted headache history. Because analgesic rebound headache assumes many of the characteristics of the underlying primary headache, diagnosis can be confusing in the absence of a careful medication history, including specific questions regarding over-the-counter headache medications and analgesics. Any change in a previously stable headache pattern needs to be taken seriously and should not automatically be attributed to analgesic overuse without a careful reevaluation of the patient.

TREATMENT

Treatment of analgesic rebound headache consists of first educating the patient about the risks of medication overuse, then discontinuation of the overused or abused drugs, and then complete abstention of the overused or abused drug or drugs for at least 3 months (Fig. 6.3). The addition of an appropriate prophylactic

MoA with MOH   MoA without MOH   MwA without MOH

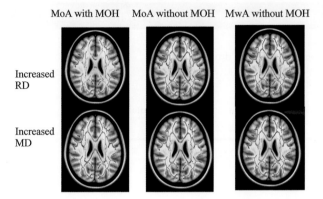

Fig. 6.2 Comparison between control and migraine without aura with medication overuse headache *(left)*, migraine with aura without medication overuse headache *(middle)*, and migraine with aura without medication overuse headache *(right)* on the whole-brain TBSS (Tract Based Spatial Statistics) skeleton. Significant increased radial diffusivity was shown in many tracts passing through the corpus callosum and the bilateral optic radiation *(upper)*. Significant increased mean diffusivity as shown in the corpus callosum *(lower)*. *Moa,* Migraine without aura; *MwA,* migraine with aura; *MOH,* medication overuse headache; *MD,* mean diffusivity. (From Shibata Y, Ishiyama S, Matsushita A. White matter diffusion abnormalities in migraine and medication overuse headache: a 1.5-T tract-based spatial statistics study. *Clin Neurol Neurosurg.* 2018;174:167–173 [Fig. 2]. ISSN 0303-8467, https://doi.org/10.1016/j.clineuro.2018.09.022, http://www.sciencedirect.com/science/article/pii/S0303846718303846)

headache treatment (e.g., propranolol for the migraineur) may further decrease the incidence of headaches in patients suffering from analgesic rebound headache (Fig. 6.4). Care should be taken to avoid abrupt discontinuation of medications such as the barbiturates and/or opioids because significant side effects, including seizures and acute abstinence syndrome, may occur. In this setting, tapering of the offending medication is necessary and may require hospitalization. Many patients cannot tolerate outpatient discontinuation of these medications and ultimately require hospitalization in a specialized headache unit. If outpatient treatment is being considered, the following points should be carefully explained to the patient:

- The headaches and associated symptoms will get worse before they get better.
- Any use, no matter how small, of the offending medications will result in continued analgesic rebound headaches.
- The patient cannot self-medicate with over-the-counter drugs.
- The significant overuse of opioids or combination medications containing butalbital or ergotamine can result in physical dependence, and discontinuation of such drugs must be done under the supervision of a physician familiar with the treatment of physical dependencies.
- If the patient follows the physician's orders regarding discontinuation of the offending medications, then the headaches can be expected to improve.

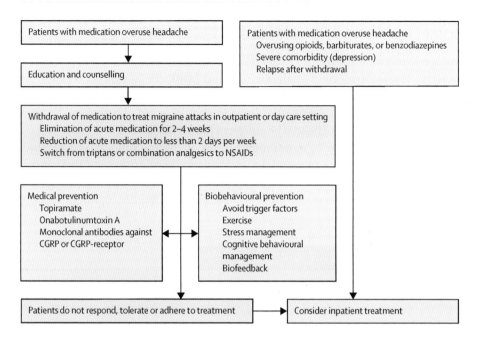

Fig. 6.3 Treatment algorithm for medication overuse headache. *CGRP*, Calcitonin gene-related peptide; *NSAIDs*, nonsteroidal antiinflammatory drugs. (Reprinted with permission from Elsevier (From Diener H-C, Dodick D, Evers S, et al. Pathophysiology, prevention, and treatment of medication overuse headache. *Lancet Neurol.* 2019;18 (9):891−902 [Fig. 1]. ISSN 1474-4422).)

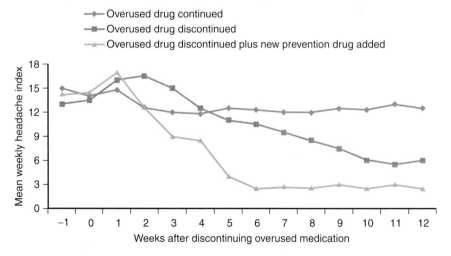

Fig. 6.4 Treatment of analgesic rebound headache consists of discontinuation of the overused or abused drugs and complete abstention of the overused or abused drug or drugs for at least 3 months. The addition of an appropriate prophylactic headache treatment (e.g., propranolol for the migraineur) may further decrease the incidence of headaches in patients suffering from medication overuse headache. (Redrawn from Mathew NT, Kurman R, Perez F. Drug induced refractory headache—clinical features and management. *Headache.* 1990;30(10):634−638, Figure 1.)

COMPLICATIONS AND PITFALLS

Analgesic rebound headache occurs much more commonly than was previously thought. The occurrence of analgesic rebound headache is a direct result of the overprescribing of abortive headache medications in patients for whom they are inappropriate. When in doubt, the clinician should avoid abortive medications altogether and treat most headache sufferers prophylactically.

Patients who overuse or abuse medications, including opioids, ergotamines, and butalbital, develop a physical dependence on these drugs, and their abrupt cessation results in a drug abstinence syndrome that can be life threatening if it is not properly treated. Therefore most of these patients require inpatient tapering in a controlled setting.

HIGH-YIELD TAKEAWAYS

- The patient is afebrile, making an acute infectious etiology unlikely.
- The patient's headaches are bilateral, making a diagnosis of migraine or cluster headache unlikely.
- The character of the patient's headache pain is neither sharp nor throbbing.
- The patient does not experience other neurologic symptoms such as weakness or speech disturbance associated with her headaches.
- The patient does not have significant photophobia and nausea and vomiting associated with her headaches.
- The patient is not experiencing significant disability associated with her headaches.
- The patient's MRI is negative.
- There are no red flags.

Suggested Readings

Abrams BM. Medication overuse headaches. *Med Clin North Am.* 2013;97(2):337–352.

Calabresi P, Cupini LM. Medication-overuse headache: similarities with drug addiction. *Trends Pharmacol Sci.* 2005;26(2):62–68.

Diener H-C, Dodick D, Evers S, et al. Pathophysiology, prevention, and treatment of medication overuse headache. *Lancet Neurol.* 2019;18(9):891–902.

Jay GW, Barkin RL. Primary headache disorders—part 2: tension-type headache and medication overuse headache. *Dis Month.* 2017;63(12):342–367.

Lau CI, Liu M-N, Chen W-H, et al. Clinical and biobehavioral perspectives: is medication overuse headache a behavior of dependence? In: Wang S-J, Lau CI, eds. *Progress in Brain Research.* Philadelphia: Elsevier; 2020:255:371–340 (chapter 14).

Michultka DM, Blanchard EB, Appelbaum KA, et al. The refractory headache patient. II. High medication consumption (analgesic rebound) headache. *Behav Res Ther.* 1989;27(4):411–420.

Moore AR, Derry S, Wiffen PJ, et al. Evidence for efficacy of acute treatment of episodic tension-type headache: methodological critique of randomised trials for oral treatments. *Pain*. 2014;155(11):2220–2228.

Ready DM. Too much of a good thing: medication overuse headache. In: Diamond S, ed. *Headache and Migraine Biology and Management*. San Diego: Academic Press; 2015: 253–266.

Rojo E, Pedraza MI, Muñoz I, et al. Chronic migraine with and without medication overuse: experience in a hospital series of 434 patients. *Neurología* (English Edition). 2015;30(3):153–157.

Shibata Y, Ishiyama S, Matsushita A. White matter diffusion abnormalities in migraine and medication overuse headache: a 1.5-T tract-based spatial statistics study. *Clin Neurol Neurosurg*. 2018;174:167–173.

Waldman SD. Analgesic rebound headache. In: *Atlas of Common Pain Syndromes*. ed. 4. Philadelphia: Elsevier; 2019:22–24.

Waldman SD. Analgesic rebound headache. In: *Pain Review*. ed. 2. Philadelphia: Elsevier; 2017:219–220.

Waldman SD. Cervical epidural block: translaminar approach. In: *Atlas of Interventional Pain Management*. ed. 5. Philadelphia: Elsevier; 2021:206–215.

Waldman SD. Targeted headache history. *Med Clin North Am*. 2013;97(2):185–195.

Westergaard ML, Glümer C, Hansen EH, et al. Prevalence of chronic headache with and without medication overuse: associations with socioeconomic position and physical and mental health status. *Pain*. 2014;155(10):2005–2013.

Yuan X, Jiang W, Ren X, et al. Predictors of relapse in patients with medication overuse headache in Shanghai: a retrospective study with a 6-month follow-up. *J Clin Neurosci*. 2019;70:33–36.

Christy Stierwalt

A 28-Year-Old Librarian With Postdural Headache Following an Epidural Block for Vaginal Delivery

- Learn the common types of headache.
- Understand the difference between primary and secondary headaches.
- Develop an understanding of clinical presentation of specific headache types.
- Develop an understanding of the treatment of specific headache types.
- Develop an understanding of the differential diagnosis of postdural headache.
- Learn how to identify factors that cause concern.

Christy Stierwalt

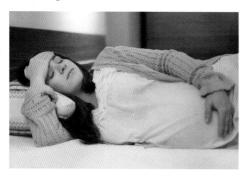

Christy Stierwalt is a 28-year-old librarian who is a gravida 2, para 2 with the chief complaint of, "Every time I sit up it feels like my head is going to explode." Christy was lying flat on the examination table with a pillow under her feet when I entered the room. She tried to sit up but immediately grabbed her head, lay back down and said, "Sorry, Doctor, the pain is just too bad when I try to sit up." Christy went on to say that as long as she stayed lying flat, she was fine, but as soon as she sat up to nurse or got up to the bathroom, her entire head starting pounding. The longer she stayed up, the worse the headache got, and then she got really nauseated. "Doctor, I apologize for my appearance. I haven't been able to wash my hair or clean up since I delivered. I know I must look a mess." I reassured her that she looked fine and that we were going to figure out what was going on and get her better so she could enjoy her beautiful new baby. I asked if there were any problems with the delivery, and Christy shook her head and said that other than being really numb for a long time after she delivered, it was a piece of cake. She volunteered that she didn't remember being that numb with her first epidural, but the numbness went away and then the headaches started. She said that the nurse told her to drink a lot of fluids and try to lie flat and that the headaches would go away. She said she drank a lot of fluids, but that made her get up to go to the bathroom, and getting up caused the headaches. "Kind of a vicious cycle, don't you think, Doctor? I can't just stay in bed! My mom came to help, but she can't miss much more work, and my husband travels. I really need to get rid of these headaches."

I asked Christy if she had any other symptoms that went along with the headache and she said that other than the nausea, there was nothing else but the headache. I asked Christy if she had identified anything that triggered her headache and she immediately answered, "Anytime I try to get up. And I mean *anytime*. There is no break, just trying to sit up a little to nurse and my head is killing me." I asked if she had any fever or stiff neck and she shook her head no.

I asked her what made it better and she said, "Pain meds do absolutely nothing but upset my stomach. As long as I lie flat, I am fine, but drinking fluids, a glass of wine, caffeine, nothing else helps at all."

I asked Christy to use one finger to point at the spot where it hurt the most. She said there was nothing to point at when she was lying flat, but if she sat up, it was her entire head. I asked her what the pain was like: an ache, sharp, stabbing, pounding, burning? She immediately said, "Pounding. It feels like my head is going to explode. The worst throbbing you can imagine, and if I don't lie down, it just gets worse and worse." I asked Christy from the time that she sat up, how long was it until she started having headache pain. She said, "It's almost immediate, and it worsens very quickly if I don't lie right back down."

On physical examination, Christy was afebrile. Her respirations were 16 and her pulse was 78 and regular. Her blood pressure was 126/80. Fundoscopic examination was normal, but Christy had an obvious sixth cranial nerve palsy on the left (Fig. 7.1). I asked if she had noticed anything funny going on with her eyes, and she said that her husband had said the headaches were making her "cross-eyed," but she thought he was just kidding around. There were no other cranial nerve abnormalities, and the remainder of her head, eyes, ears, nose throat (HEENT) examination was completely normal. Her cervical paraspinous muscles were mildly tender, but no myofascial trigger points were identified. Her cardiopulmonary examination was normal, as was her thyroid. Her abdominal examination revealed no abnormal mass or

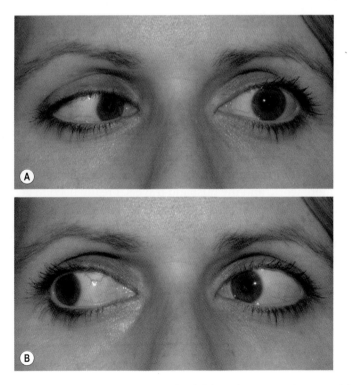

Fig. 7.1 (A) Idiopathic left sixth nerve palsy causing left lateral rectus weakness and limitation of abduction in a young adult. (B) Conjugate gaze to the right is normal. (From Liu G, Volpe N, Galetta S, et al. *Galetta's Neuro-Ophthalmology.* ed. 3. New York: Elsevier; 2019 [Fig. 15.37a-b].)

organomegaly, and there was no rebound tenderness present. There was no costovertebral angle (CVA) tenderness. There was no peripheral edema. A careful neurologic examination of the upper and lower extremities revealed no evidence of weakness, lack of coordination, or peripheral or entrapment neuropathy, and her deep tendon reflexes were normal. Christy's mental status exam was within normal limits. I asked Christy to try and sit up, which immediately triggered her headache, so I put her flat. I told her that I was pretty sure I knew what was going on, and the good news was there was an easy fix to get rid of her headaches. She smiled and said, "That's why you get paid the big bucks!"

Key Clinical Points—What's Important and What's Not
THE HISTORY

- Recent onset of postdural headache following an epidural block for vaginal delivery
- Headache occurs when patient moves from supine to sitting position
- Headache resolves when patient returns to supine position
- Headaches are holocranial
- Character of the headache pain is throbbing
- Patient denies fever or chills
- Patient notes the onset of nausea if remaining in the upright position
- Significant disability associated with headache; specifically, patient is unable to care for her newborn

THE PHYSICAL EXAMINATION

- Patient is afebrile
- Normal fundoscopic exam
- Left sixth cranial nerve palsy is noted
- Neurologic exam is otherwise normal
- Headache triggered by moving patient from supine to sitting position

OTHER FINDINGS OF NOTE

- Normal cardiovascular examination
- Normal pulmonary examination
- Normal abdominal examination
- No peripheral edema
- Normal upper and lower extremity neurologic examination, motor and sensory examination

What Tests Would You Like to Order?

The following tests were ordered:
- No tests were ordered.

TEST RESULTS

None

 Clinical Correlation—Putting It All Together

What is the diagnosis?
Postdural puncture headache

The Science Behind the Diagnosis

CLINICAL SYNDROME

When the dura is intentionally or accidentally punctured, the potential for head-ache exists. The clinical presentation of postdural puncture headache is classic and makes the diagnosis straightforward if considering this diagnostic category of headache. The diagnosis may be obscured if the clinician is unaware that dural puncture may have occurred, or in the rare instance when this type of headache occurs spontaneously after a bout of sneezing or coughing. The symptoms and rare physical findings associated with postdural puncture headache are due to low cerebrospinal fluid pressure resulting from continued leakage of spinal fluid out of the subarachnoid space.

The symptoms of postdural puncture headache begin almost immediately after the patient moves from a horizontal to an upright position (Fig. 7.2). The intensity peaks within 1 or 2 minutes and abates within several minutes of the patient again assuming the horizontal position. The headache is pounding in character, and its intensity is severe, with the intensity increasing the longer the patient remains upright. The headache is almost always bilateral and located in the frontotemporal, and occipital regions. Nausea, vomiting, and dizziness frequently accompany the headache pain, especially if the patient remains upright. The headache gradually resolves within 30 minutes of the patient resuming the supine position.

SIGNS AND SYMPTOMS

The diagnosis of postdural puncture headache is most often made on the basis of clinical history rather than physical findings on examination. The neurologic

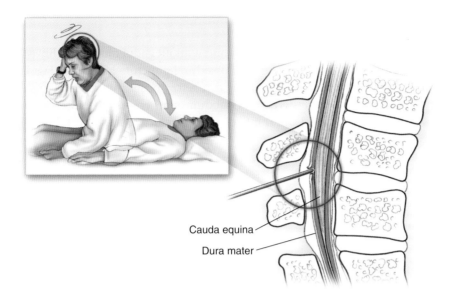

Cauda equina
Dura mater

Fig. 7.2 The onset of headache that occurs when the patient moves from the horizontal to the upright position is the sine qua non of postdural puncture headache. (From Waldman S. *Atlas of Uncommon Pain Syndromes*. ed. 3. Philadelphia: Elsevier; 2020 [Fig. 13-1]. 9780323640770.)

examination in most patients suffering from postdural puncture headache is normal. If the spinal fluid leak is allowed to persist or if the patient remains in the upright position for long periods despite the headache, cranial nerve palsies may occur, with the sixth cranial nerve affected most commonly (see Fig. 7.1). This complication may be transient, but it may become permanent, especially in patients with vulnerable nerves, such as those with diabetes. If the neurologic examination is abnormal, other causes of headache should be considered, including subarachnoid hemorrhage.

The onset of headache pain and other associated symptoms, such as nausea and vomiting, that occur when the patient moves from the horizontal to the upright position and then abate when the patient resumes a horizontal position is the sine qua non of postdural puncture headache (see Fig. 7.2). A history of intentional dural puncture, such as lumbar puncture, spinal anesthesia or myelography, or accidental dural puncture, such as failed epidural block or dural injury during spinal surgery, strongly points to the diagnosis of postdural puncture headache. As mentioned, a spontaneous postdural headache that manifests identically to headache after dural puncture can occur after bouts of heavy sneezing or coughing and is thought to be due to traumatic rents in the dura. In this setting, a diagnosis of postdural puncture headache is one of exclusion.

TESTING

Magnetic resonance imaging (MRI) with and without gadolinium is highly accurate in helping confirm the diagnosis of postdural puncture headache (Fig. 7.3). Enhancement of the dura with low-lying cerebellar tonsils invariably is present. Poor visualization of the cisterns and subdural and epidural fluid collections also may be identified, and dural infoldings secondary to loss of cerebrospinal fluid may be identified.

No additional testing is indicated for a patient who has undergone dural puncture and then develops a classic postdural headache, unless infection or subarachnoid hemorrhage is suspected. In this setting, lumbar puncture, complete blood cell count, and erythrocyte sedimentation rate are indicated on an emergent basis.

DIFFERENTIAL DIAGNOSIS

If the clinician is aware that the patient has undergone dural puncture, the diagnosis of postdural puncture headache is usually made. Delayed diagnosis most often occurs in settings in which dural puncture is not suspected.

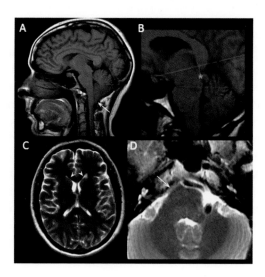

Fig. 7.3 Persistent untreated postdural puncture headache. Magnetic resonance imaging of the head showing cerebrospinal fluid hypotension. (A) Descent of the cerebellar tonsils below the foramen magnum *(arrow)*. (B) Iter *(asterisk)* is below the incisural line *(green line)*. (C) Presence of ventricular collapse *(arrows)*. (D) Obliteration of the preopontine cistern *(arrow)*. (From Villamil F, Ruella M, Perez A, et al. Traumatic vs spontaneous cerebrospinal fluid hypotension headache: our experience in a series of 137 cases. *Clin Neurol Neurosurg*. 2020;198:106—140 [Fig. 2]. ISSN 0303-8467, https://doi.org/10.1016/j.clineuro.2020.106140, http://www.sciencedirect.com/science/article/pii/S0303846720304832)

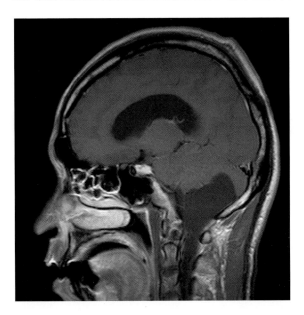

Fig. 7.4 Magnetic resonance imaging of head showing a giant infracerebellar arachnoid cyst herniating below the level of the foramen magnum. (From Lu K-C, Chao C-C, Wang T-L, et al. A differential diagnosis in postural headache: herniation of a giant posterior fossa arachnoid cyst. *Am J Emerg Med*. 2008;26 (2):247.e1−247.e3 [Fig. 1]. ISSN 0735-6757, https://doi.org/10.1016/j.ajem.2007.04.005, http://www.sciencedirect.com/science/article/pii/S0735675707002677)

Occasionally, postdural puncture headache is misdiagnosed as migraine headache because of the associated nausea and vomiting coupled with visual disturbance. In any patient with dural puncture, infection remains an ever-present possibility. If fever is present, immediate lumbar puncture and blood cultures should be obtained and the patient started on antibiotics that cover resistant strains of Staphylococcus. MRI to rule out epidural abscess also should be considered if fever is present. Subarachnoid hemorrhage may mimic postdural puncture headache, but it should be identified on MRI of the brain. Rarely, other causes of postdural headache can mimic the presentation of postdural puncture headache and must be considered in the differential diagnosis, especially in the parturient (Fig. 7.4, Tables 7.1 and 7.2).

TREATMENT

The mainstay of treatment of postdural puncture headache is the administration of autologous blood into the epidural space (Fig. 7.5). This technique is known as epidural blood patch and is highly successful in the treatment of

TABLE 7.1 ■ Causes of Postdural Headache

- Intentional dural puncture
- Inadvertent dural puncture
- Spontaneous intracranial hypotension
- Dural rents following sneezing or heavy lifting
- Dural tears during spine surgery
- Cerebrospinal fluid fistula
- Cerebrospinal fluid shunt over drainage
- Type 1 Arnold-Chiari malformation
- Colloid cysts of the third ventricle
- Cerebellar hemorrhage
- Superior sagittal sinus thrombosis
- Arachnoid cysts of the posterior fossa

TABLE 7.2 ■ Differential Diagnosis of Postpartum Headache

Postdural puncture headache
Preeclampsia
Space-occupying lesion
Dehydration
Withdrawal from illicit substances
Meningitis
Abscess
Encephalitis
Sinusitis
Ischemic stroke
Intracranial hemorrhage
Venous sinus thrombosis
Vasculitis
Migraine with or without aura
Tension-type headache
Cluster (very rare in females; must be considered a diagnosis of exclusion)

postdural puncture headache. A volume of 12 to 18 mL of autologous blood is injected slowly into the epidural space at the level of dural puncture under strict aseptic precautions (Fig. 7.6). The patient should remain in the horizontal position for the next 12 to 24 hours. Relief occurs within 2 to 3 hours in more than 90% of patients. Approximately 10% of patients experience temporary relief and then a recurrence of symptoms when assuming the upright position. These patients should undergo a second epidural blood patch within 24 hours. If the patient has experienced significant nausea and vomiting, antiemetics combined with intravenous fluids help speed recovery. Some clinicians have advocated the use of alcoholic beverages to suppress the secretion of antidiuretic hormone and increase cerebrospinal fluid production. Caffeine

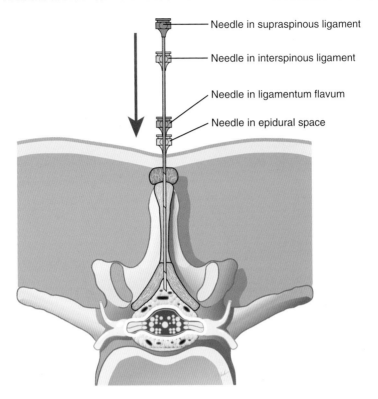

Needle in supraspinous ligament

Needle in interspinous ligament

Needle in ligamentum flavum

Needle in epidural space

Fig. 7.5 Anatomy of the epidural and subarachnoid space. (From Waldman S. *Atlas of Interventional Pain Management*. ed. 5. Philadelphia: Elsevier; 2021 [Fig. 107.5].)

also has been reported to be helpful in treating the headache pain. There are also anecdotal reports that the use of high-concentration oxygen combined with administration of metoclopramide may palliate the pain of postdural puncture headache in patients with a contraindication to epidural blood patch.

COMPLICATIONS AND PITFALLS

The diagnosis of postdural puncture headache is made by obtaining a thorough, targeted headache history and performing a careful physical examination. The postdural nature is pathognomonic for postdural puncture headache, and its presence should lead the clinician to strongly consider the diagnosis of postdural puncture headache. The incidence of postdural puncture headache after lumbar puncture, myelography, or spinal anesthesia can be decreased by using needles with a smaller diameter and placing

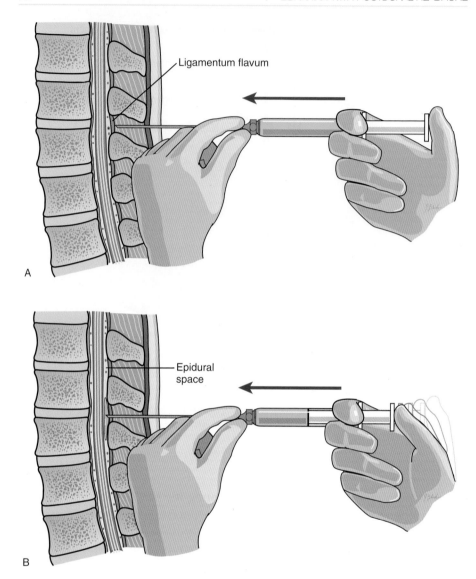

Fig. 7.6   Identification of the lumbar epidural space using the loss of resistance technique to perform epidural blood patch. (From Waldman S. *Atlas of Interventional Pain Management*. ed. 5. Philadelphia: Elsevier; 2021 [Fig. 107.9].)

the needle bevel parallel to the dural fibers (Fig. 7.7). Special noncutting needles may decrease further the incidence of postdural puncture headache.

Failure to recognize, diagnose, and treat postdural puncture headache promptly may result in considerable pain and suffering for the patient. If the low

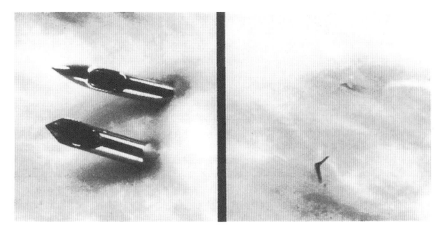

Fig. 7.7 Comparison of dural puncture holes made by Quincke and Sprotte needles. The Sprotte atraumatic needle is above the cutting Quincke needle. (From Sladky JH, Piwinski SE. Lumbar puncture technique and lumbar drains. *Atlas Oral Maxillofac Surg Clin.* 2015;23(2):169–176 [Fig. 2].)

cerebrospinal fluid pressure is allowed to persist, cranial nerve deficits may occur. In most instances, the cranial nerve deficits are temporary, but in rare instances, these deficits may become permanent, especially in patients with vulnerable nerves, such as those with diabetes. MRI of the brain is indicated in all patients thought to be suffering from headaches associated with dural puncture. Failure to diagnose central nervous system infection correctly can result in significant mortality and morbidity.

HIGH-YIELD TAKEAWAYS

- The patient is afebrile, making an acute infectious etiology unlikely.
- The patient's headache is postdural, and it began following an epidural block to provide analgesia for vaginal delivery.
- The headache occurs when patient moves from the supine to the upright position.
- The headache resolves when the patient returns to the supine position.
- Untreated postdural puncture headache can result in cranial nerve palsies.
- The patient is experiencing significant disability associated with her headaches.

Suggested Readings

Haller G, Cornet J, Boldi M-O, et al. Risk factors for post-dural puncture headache following injury of the dural membrane: a root-cause analysis and nested case-control study. *Int J Obstetr Anesth.* 2018;36:17–27.

Panigrahi AR, Armstrong C. Post-dural puncture headache in the parturient. *Anaesth Intens Care Med*. 2019;20(9):470–473.

Russell R, Laxton C, Lucas DN, et al. Treatment of obstetric post-dural puncture headache. Part 1: conservative and pharmacological management. *Int J Obstetr Anesth*. 2019;38:93–103.

Russell R, Laxton C, Lucas DN, et al. Treatment of obstetric post-dural puncture headache. Part 2: epidural blood patch. *Int J Obstetr Anesth*. 2019;38:104–118.

Spring A, McMorrow R. Successful treatment of a recurrent post-dural puncture headache with an epidural blood patch 18 months after the initial dural puncture. *Int J Obstetr Anesth*. 2019;40:152–153.

Waldman SD. Post-dural puncture headache. In: *Atlas of Uncommon Pain Syndromes*. ed. 4. Philadelphia: Elsevier; 2021:40–42.

Waldman SD. Targeted headache history. *Med Clin North Am*. 2013;97(2):185–195.

Waldman SD, Feldstein GS, Allen ML. Cervical epidural blood patch for treatment of cervical dural puncture headache. *Anesth Rev*. 1987;14:23–25.

Amy Lin

A 46-Year-Old Female With Posttraumatic Occipital Headaches

- Develop an understanding of the causes of occipital neuralgia.
- Learn the clinical presentation of occipital neuralgia.
- Learn how to use physical examination to help diagnose occipital neuralgia.
- Learn to distinguish occipital neuralgia from tension-type headache.
- Learn the important anatomic structures in occipital neuralgia.
- Develop an understanding of the treatment options for occipital neuralgia.
- Learn the appropriate testing options to help diagnose occipital neuralgia.
- Learn to identify red flags in patients who present with occipital neuralgia.
- Develop an understanding of the role in interventional pain management in the treatment of occipital neuralgia.

Amy Lin

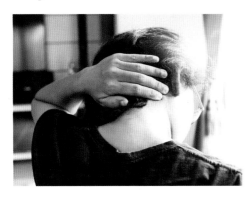

"He hit me right in the back of my head," bemoaned Amy Lin. Amy had been my patient since moving to the city a couple of years ago. A successful nail salon owner, Amy seemed to have it all together. I had seen Amy for an upper respiratory tract infection about 8 months ago, but other than that, she was pretty healthy. Amy had called the office earlier in the week and asked if we could work her in because she had a pain in the back of her head that just refused to get better.

"Doctor, you know that husband of mine, Joe, is always getting hurt? Well, this time he decided to take it out on me." Amy went on to say that about 3 weeks ago, she wanted to knock down a bird's nest that was in the gutter over her patio door, so she asked Joe to get the ladder out for her. She was walking behind Joe as he carried the ladder, and when he suddenly turned, the ladder hit Amy squarely on the back of her head. "Doc, he really rang my bell! I saw stars, and it brought tears to my eyes. I gave him what-for and grabbed the ladder away from him before he killed me with it. I got the bird's nest down, but for the past 3 weeks, the back of my head has been killing me. I've tried to tough it out. I tried all the usual stuff: tea tree oil, Motrin, the heating pad. Joe wanted me to go to the chiropractor, but I was afraid it might make my head worse. I think it's about time to trade Joe in on a new and improved model." I could tell that Amy was getting really wound up about Joe, so I reassured her that she had done every-thing right, except perhaps letting Joe carry the ladder. I asked her if she had ever had headaches before and she shook her head no. "So, no loss of conscious-ness?" and again she shook her head no. I suggested that we look her over to figure out what was wrong and what we could do to make it better.

I asked Amy to point with one finger where it hurt the most. Amy pointed to her left occipital region, and then pointed up toward the vertex of her scalp. "Is there any numbness?" I asked. Amy replied that the left side of her head felt like it was asleep. "You know, Doctor, that weird pins-and-needles feeling that you get when your foot goes to sleep."

"Are you having any visual problems, or is there anything else that I need to know about?" I asked.

"Nothing but my husband, Joe. He means well, but he is always an accident waiting to happen."

"Let's put you in a gown and take a look," I said.

On physical examination, Amy was afebrile and her respirations were 16. Her pulse was 74 and regular, her blood pressure a nice 110/68. Palpation of her cranium revealed no mass or other abnormality. Her head, eyes, ears, nose, throat (HEENT) exam, including fundoscopic examination, was normal, as was her cardiopulmonary examination. Her abdominal examination revealed no abnormal mass or organomegaly. There was no costovertebral angle (CVA) tenderness. There was no peripheral edema. Palpation over the left greater and lesser occipital nerves elicited a shocklike pain that radiated from the nuchal ridge to the top of her head on the left. Her neurologic examination was otherwise within normal limits. There were no pathologic reflexes.

Given the history of trauma, I ordered a magnetic resonance imaging (MRI) of the brain to rule out any occult pathology.

Key Clinical Points—What's Important and What's Not

THE HISTORY

- History of acute trauma to the left occiput when hit with a ladder
- No loss of consciousness
- No history of previous headache
- Headache is located primarily in the left occipital region with pain radiating to vertex of the scalp
- A pins-and-needles sensation in the distribution of the pain

THE PHYSICAL EXAMINATION

- Patient is afebrile
- Tenderness over the greater and lesser occipital nerve
- Deep palpation over the greater and lesser occipital nerve reproduces the neuritic pain that radiates to the vertex of the scalp
- Normal fundoscopic examination
- Normal neurologic examination, upper extremity motor and sensory examination
- No pathologic reflexes

OTHER FINDINGS OF NOTE

- Normal HEENT examination
- Normal cardiovascular examination
- Normal pulmonary examination
- Normal abdominal examination
- No peripheral edema

What Tests Would You Like to Order?

The following tests were ordered:
- MRI of the brain

TEST RESULTS

The MRI of the brain was normal.

 Clinical Correlation—Putting It All Together

What is the diagnosis?
Occipital neuralgia

The Science Behind the Diagnosis

CLINICAL SYNDROME

Occipital neuralgia is usually the result of blunt trauma to the greater and lesser occipital nerves (Fig. 8.1). The greater occipital nerve arises from fibers of the dorsal primary ramus of the second cervical nerve and, to a lesser extent, from fibers of the third cervical nerve. The greater occipital nerve pierces the fascia just below the superior nuchal ridge, along with the occipital artery. It supplies the medial portion of the posterior scalp as far anterior as the vertex (see Fig. 8.1). The lesser occipital nerve arises from the ventral primary rami of the second and third cervical nerves. The lesser occipital nerve passes superiorly along the posterior border of the sternocleidomastoid muscle and divides into cutaneous branches that innervate the lateral portion of the posterior scalp and the cranial surface of the pinna of the ear (Fig. 8.2).

Less commonly, repetitive microtrauma from working with the neck hyperextended (e.g., painting ceilings) or looking for prolonged periods at a computer monitor whose focal point is too high, thus extending the cervical spine, may also cause occipital neuralgia. Occipital neuralgia is characterized by persistent pain at the base of the skull with occasional sudden, shocklike paresthesias in the distribution of the greater and lesser occipital nerves. Tension-type headache, which is much more common, occasionally mimics the pain of occipital neuralgia.

SIGNS AND SYMPTOMS

A patient suffering from occipital neuralgia experiences neuritic pain in the distribution of the greater and lesser occipital nerves when the nerves are palpated at the level of the nuchal ridge. Some patients can elicit pain with rotation or

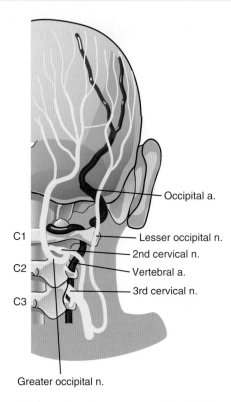

C1

C2

C3

Occipital a.

Lesser occipital n.

2nd cervical n.

Vertebral a.

3rd cervical n.

Greater occipital n.

Fig. 8.1 Anatomy of the occipital nerves. *a*, Artery; *n*, nerve. (From Waldman S. *Atlas of Interventional Pain Management*. ed. 5. Philadelphia: Elsevier; 2021 [Fig. 7.1].)

lateral bending of the cervical spine. Deep palpation of the greater and lesser occipital nerves may also elicit pain.

TESTING

No specific test exists for occipital neuralgia. Testing is aimed primarily at identifying an occult pathologic process or other diseases that may mimic occipital neuralgia (see "Differential Diagnosis"). All patients with the recent onset of headache or head trauma thought to be occipital neuralgia should undergo MRI of the brain and cervical spine. MRI should also be performed in patients with previously stable occipital neuralgia who have experienced a recent change in headache symptoms (Fig. 8.3). Computed tomography (CT) scanning of the brain and cervical spine may also be useful in identifying intracranial disease that may mimic the symptoms of occipital neuralgia (Fig. 8.4). Screening laboratory tests consisting of a complete blood count, erythrocyte sedimentation rate, and automated blood chemistry should be performed if the diagnosis of occipital neuralgia is in question.

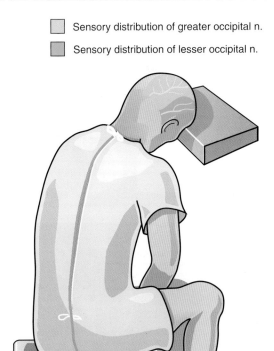

☐ Sensory distribution of greater occipital n.

☐ Sensory distribution of lesser occipital n.

Fig. 8.2 The sensory distribution of the greater and lesser occipital nerve. *n*, Nerve. (From Waldman S. *Atlas of Interventional Pain Management*. ed. 5. Philadelphia: Elsevier; 2021 [Fig. 7.2].)

DIFFERENTIAL DIAGNOSIS

Occipital neuralgia is an infrequent cause of headache and rarely occurs in the absence of trauma to the greater and lesser occipital nerves. More often, patients with headaches involving the occipital region are suffering from tension-type headache. Tension-type headache does not respond to occipital nerve blocks but is amenable to treatment with antidepressants, such as amitriptyline, in conjunction with cervical epidural nerve block. Rarely, other pathologic processes may mimic the clinical presentation of occipital neuralgia (Table 8.1). Therefore the clinician should reconsider the diagnosis of occipital neuralgia in patients whose symptoms are consistent with occipital neuralgia but who fail to respond to greater and lesser occipital nerve blocks.

TREATMENT

The treatment of occipital neuralgia consists primarily of neural blockade with local anesthetic and steroid, combined with the judicious use of nonsteroidal

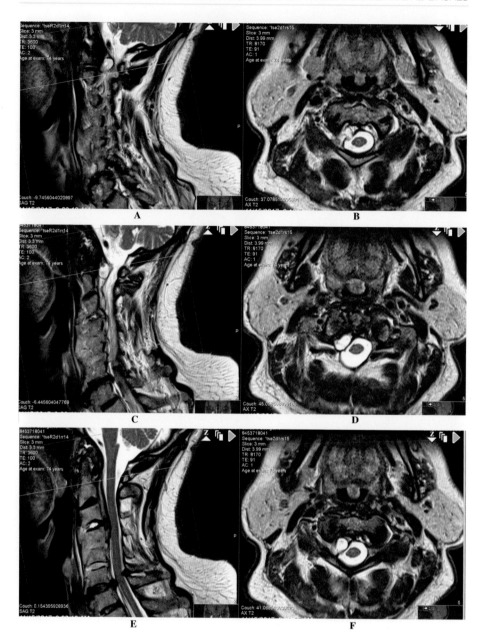

Fig. 8.3   (A—F) Magnetic resonance imaging scan of a patient with a clinical diagnosis of occipital neuralgia. T2 sequences with sagittal (A, C, E) and axial (B, D, F) views of cervical spine depicting the T2 hyperintense cyst (synovial) of right-sided C1-C2 facet joint with compression of the C2 nerve root and its ganglion. (E) There appears to be C6-C7 focal disc herniation with mild compression at the index level. However, the patient was not symptomatic from this level. (From Janjua MJ, Reddy S, El Ahmadieh TY, et al. Occipital neuralgia: a neurosurgical perspective. *J Clin Neurosci.* 2020;71:263—270 [Fig. 4]. ISSN 0967-5868, https://doi.org/10.1016/j.jocn.2019.08.102, http://www.sciencedirect.com/science/article/pii/S0967586819314110)

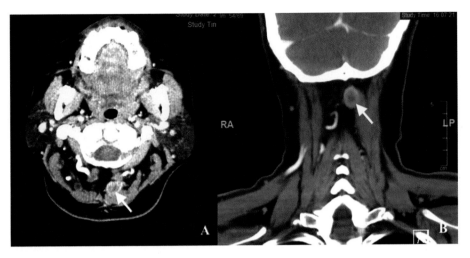

Fig. 8.4 Computed tomography neck axial (A) and coronal (B) images showing a hypodense rim-enhancing lesion in the left occipital region. (From Lee SYC, Lim MY, Loke SC, et al. Greater occipital nerve schwannoma—a rare cause of occipital neuralgia. *Otolaryngol Case Rep*. 2020;14:100143 [Fig. 2]. ISSN 2468-5488, https://doi.org/10.1016/j.xocr.2019.100143, http://www.sciencedirect.com/science/article/pii/S2468548819300736.)

TABLE 8.1 ■ Differential Diagnosis of Occipital Neuralgia

Tension-type headache
Rheumatoid arthritis involving the upper cervical facet joints
Osteoarthritis involving the upper cervical facet joints
Arnold-Chiari malformation
Acceleration-deceleration injuries
Iatrogenic damage to the occipital nerves
Atlantoaxial subluxation
Atlantoaxial lateral masses
C2-C3 radiculopathy
C2-C3 subluxation or arthropathy
Cervical myelopathy
Posterior fossa tumor
Acromegaly
Neurofibromatosis type 1
Paget disease
Giant cell arteritis
Hemicrania continua
Herpes zoster
Pott disease
Synovial facet cyst
Neuritis
Neurosyphilis

antiinflammatory drugs, muscle relaxants, tricyclic antidepressants, and physical therapy.

To perform neural blockade of the greater and lesser occipital nerves, the patient is placed in a sitting position with the cervical spine flexed and the forehead on a padded bedside table (see Fig. 8.2). A total of 8 mL of local anesthetic is drawn up in a 12-mL sterile syringe. For treatment of occipital neuralgia or other painful conditions involving the greater and lesser occipital nerves, a total of 80 mg methylprednisolone is added to the local anesthetic with the first block, and 40 mg of depot steroid is added with subsequent blocks. The occipital artery is palpated at the level of the superior nuchal ridge. After the skin is prepared with antiseptic solution, a 1.5-inch, 22-gauge needle is inserted just medial to the artery and is advanced perpendicularly until the needle approaches the periosteum of the underlying occipital bone. Paresthesias may be elicited, and the patient should be warned of this possibility. The needle is then redirected superiorly, and after gentle aspiration, 5 mL of solution is injected in a fanlike distribution with care taken to avoid the foramen magnum, which is located medially (Fig. 8.5). The lesser occipital nerve and several superficial branches of the

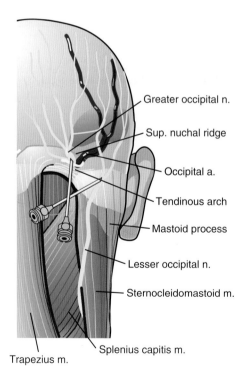

Fig. 8.5 Technique for landmark-guided occipital nerve block. *a*, Artery; *m*, muscle; *n*, nerve. (From Waldman S. *Atlas of Interventional Pain Management*. ed. 5. Philadelphia: Elsevier; 2021 [Fig. 7.3].)

greater occipital nerve are then blocked by directing the needle laterally and slightly inferiorly. After gentle aspiration, an additional 3 to 4 mL of solution is injected (see Fig. 8.5). Ultrasound needle guidance may improve the accuracy of needle placement in some patients. Should the patient experience a recurrence of symptoms after initial relief from a trial of occipital nerve blocks, radiofrequency lesioning of the affected occipital nerves is a reasonable next step (Figs. 8.6, 8.7, and 8.8). For patients suffering from occipital neuralgia that fails to respond to the foregoing treatment modalities, a trial of injection of type A botulinum toxin or occipital nerve stimulation should be considered (Fig. 8.9).

COMPLICATIONS AND PITFALLS

The most common reason that greater and lesser occipital nerve blocks fail to relieve headache pain is that the patient has been misdiagnosed. Any patient with headaches so severe that they require neural blockade should undergo MRI of the head to rule out unsuspected intracranial disease. Further, cervical spine radiographs should be considered to rule out congenital abnormalities such as Arnold-Chiari malformations that may be the hidden cause of the patient's occipital headaches.

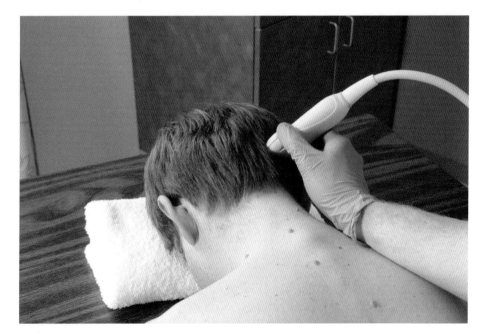

Fig. 8.6 Proper ultrasound transducer placement for greater and lesser occipital block. (Courtesy Steven D. Waldman, MD.)

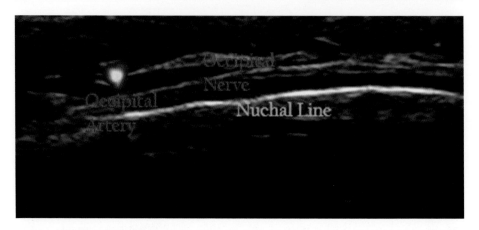

Fig. 8.7 Color Doppler image demonstrating the relationship of the occipital artery and occipital nerve. (Courtesy Steven D. Waldman, MD.)

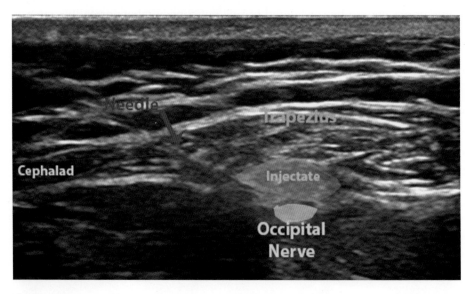

Fig. 8.8 Ultrasound-guided greater occipital nerve block. (Courtesy Steven D. Waldman, MD.)

The scalp is highly vascular. This vascularity, coupled with the close proximity to arteries of both the greater and lesser occipital nerves, means that the clinician must carefully calculate the total dose of local anesthetic that can be safely given, especially if bilateral nerve blocks are being performed. This vascularity and the proximity to the arterial supply give rise to an increased incidence of

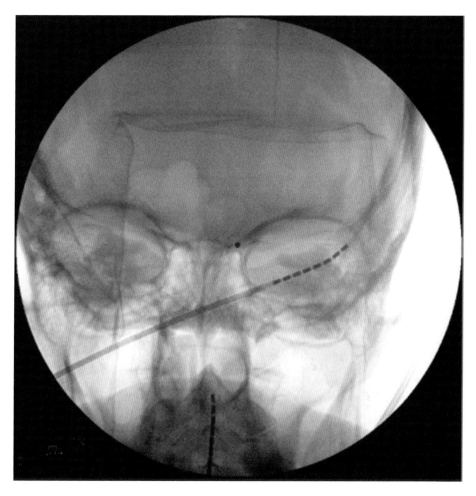

Fig. 8.9 Occipital nerve stimulation. (Courtesy Steven D. Waldman, MD.)

postblock ecchymosis and hematoma formation. These complications can be decreased if manual pressure is applied to the area of the block immediately after injection. Application of cold packs for 20 minutes after the block can also decrease the amount of pain and bleeding. Care must be taken to avoid inadvertent needle placement into the foramen magnum because the subarachnoid administration of local anesthetic in this region results in immediate total spinal anesthesia. As with other headache syndromes, the clinician must be sure that the diagnosis is correct and that the patient has no coexistent intracranial disease or disease of the cervical spine that may be erroneously attributed to occipital neuralgia.

HIGH-YIELD TAKEAWAYS

- The patient is afebrile, making an acute infectious etiology unlikely.
- The patient's symptomatology is the result of acute trauma to the greater and lesser occipital.
- The patient's pain is localized to the left occipital nerve.
- The patient's pain is in the distribution of the greater occipital nerve.
- MRI is indicated in all patients with posttraumatic headache.
- Occipital nerve block is useful in the palliation of occipital neuralgia.

Suggested Readings

Finiels P-J, Batifol D. The treatment of occipital neuralgia: review of 111 cases. *Neurochirurgie*. 2016;62(5):233–240.

Janjua MB, Reddy S, El Ahmadieh TY, et al. Occipital neuralgia: a neurosurgical perspective. *J Clin Neurosci*. 2020;71:263–270.

Lee SYC, Lim MY, Loke SC, et al. Greater occipital nerve schwannoma—a rare cause of occipital neuralgia. *Otolaryngol Case Rep*. 2020;14:100143.

Waldman SD. Greater and lesser occipital nerve block. In: *Atlas of Interventional Pain Management*. ed. 5. Philadelphia: Elsevier; 2021:27–30.

Waldman SD. Occipital neuralgia. In: *Pain Review*. ed. 2. Philadelphia: Saunders; 2017: 256–257.

Waldman SD. Occipital neuralgia. In: *Atlas of Common Pain Syndromes*. ed. 4. Philadelphia: Elsevier; 2019:25–27.

Cassandra Elliot

A 29-Year-Old Overweight Female With Constant Headache Pain That Worsens With Valsalva Maneuver

- Learn the common types of headache.
- Understand the difference between primary and secondary headaches associated with increased intracranial pressure.
- Develop an understanding of clinical presentation of specific headache types.
- Develop an understanding of the treatment of specific headache types.
- Develop an understanding of the differential diagnosis of headaches that increase with Valsalva maneuver.
- Learn the importance of fundoscopic examination in the diagnosis of headache.
- Learn how to identify factors that cause concern.

Cassandra Elliott

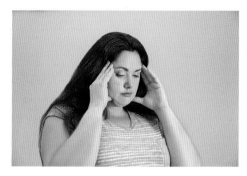

Cassandra Elliott is a 29-year-old intensive care unit nurse with the chief complaint of, "My head is killing me." Cassandra stated that over the past 4 or 5 weeks, she began noticing that shortly after awakening, she began to experience a headache that involved her entire head. Cassandra stated that the pain was constant and throbbing in nature. I asked her if she noticed anything that made the pain worse and she said, "Lifting patients up in bed and straining at stool makes it feel like the top of my head was going to blow off. Doctor, I don't mean to waste your time, but a few days ago a patient fell, and when I was helping lift him off the floor, my vision went out for a few minutes. I sat down and the sensation of looking through a tunnel gradually went away. I don't mean to sound like a wimp, but I was really scared. I know that I need to lose some weight, and I thought I was having a stroke or something. The other thing that is really worrying me is that I am having trouble reading fine print. At first I thought I just needed to get some reading glasses, but I am scared that something really bad is going on." I asked Cassandra if she had any numbness or other neurologic symptoms associated with her headache pain, and she just shook her head.

Cassandra denied any fever, chills, or other constitutional symptoms. I asked Cassandra if she had recently started any medications, specifically tetracycline, vitamin A, retinoids, danzol, or oral contraceptives, and she said no. I asked Cassandra what made her pain better, and she said that avoiding lifting or coughing seemed to help, but the use of acetaminophen and ibuprofen was of no value whatsoever. She denied significant sleep disturbance.

I asked Cassandra about any antecedent head trauma, and she just shook her head no. She volunteered, "Doctor, I am really scared. Do you think I have a brain tumor or an aneurysm or something? I've never had anything like this before. Something is definitely not right."

I asked Cassandra to point with one finger to show me where it hurt the most. She held her temples and said that her entire head hurt. "Doctor, it really hurts all the time."

On physical examination, Cassandra was afebrile. Her respirations were 18, and her pulse was 78 and regular. Her blood pressure was 130/78. Cassandra was overweight, with a body mass index (BMI) of 40. Cassandra's fundoscopic examination revealed papilledema bilaterally (Fig. 9.1). "Not good," I thought. There were no cranial nerve abnormalities, and the remainder of her ear, nose, and throat (ENT) examination was unremarkable. Her visual acuity was grossly

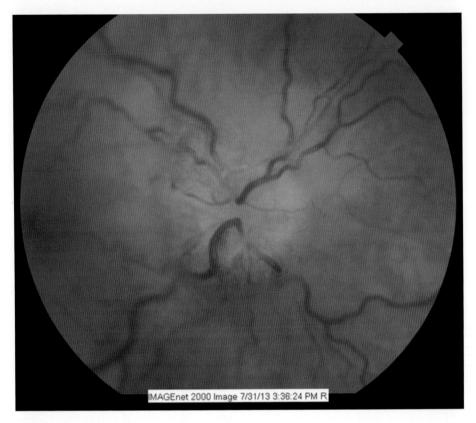

Fig. 9.1 Severe papilledema in a patient suffering from pseudotumor cerebri. (Courtesy Corey W. Waldman, MD.)

intact, but she appeared to have visual field defects. Her cardiopulmonary examination was normal. Her thyroid was normal. Her abdominal examination revealed no abnormal mass or organomegaly. There was no costovertebral angle (CVA) tenderness. There was no peripheral edema. Her low back examination was unremarkable. A careful neurologic examination revealed no evidence of peripheral neuropathy, entrapment neuropathy, or other abnormalities. Deep tendon reflexes were normal, and no pathologic reflexes were present.

Key Clinical Points—What's Important and What's Not
THE HISTORY

- Recent onset of holocranial headaches in the absence of antecedent trauma
- Headache worsened with Valsalva maneuver
- Associated visual disturbance

- Patient is very concerned about her symptoms
- No history of fever or chills
- Patient specifically denies recently starting tetracycline, vitamin A, retinoids, danzol, or oral contraceptives

THE PHYSICAL EXAMINATION

- Patient is afebrile
- Patient is female
- Patient is obese
- Bilateral papilledema present (see Fig. 9.1)
- Visual field defects identified
- No cranial nerve palsies
- Neurologic examination is normal

OTHER FINDINGS OF NOTE

- Normal ENT examination
- Normal cardiovascular examination
- Normal pulmonary examination
- Normal abdominal examination
- No peripheral edema

 What Tests Would You Like to Order?

The following tests were ordered:
- Magnetic resonance (MRI) of the brain
- Visual field testing

TEST RESULTS

MRI of the brain revealed normal brain parenchyma with no evidence of hydrocephaly, masses, structural lesions, or meningeal enhancements, but some flattening of the posterior sclera and bulging of the optic discs were noted (Figs. 9.2 and 9.3).

Visual field testing was markedly abnormal, with an abnormally enlarged blind spot and a nasal step defect affecting the inferior quadrants of the visual field (Fig. 9.4).

 Clinical Correlation—Putting It All Together

What is the diagnosis?
Pseudotumor cerebri

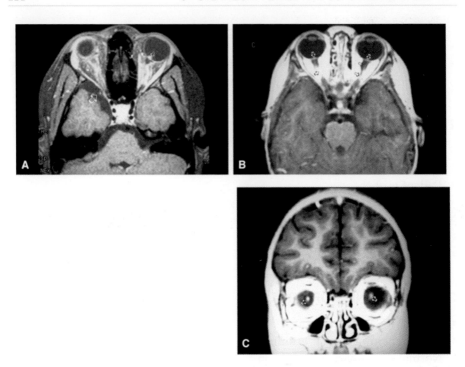

Fig. 9.2 Enhancement of the prelaminar optic nerve. A, T_1-weighted axial image (case 1) with fat suppression shows maximal prelaminar enhancement in the left eye (upper arrow). There is a probable arachnoid cyst producing a hypointense signal anterior to the right temporal lobe in the middle fossa (lower arrow). B, T_1-weighted axial image (case 3) shows prelaminar enhancement of both optic nerves (upper arrows). Also note prominent perioptic CSF (middle arrow in left orbit) and vertical tortuosity of both optic nerves with "smear sign" (lower arrows in both orbits). C, T_1-weighted coronal image showing focal enhancement of the prelaminar optic nerves within the globes (arrows). (From Michael C Brodsky, Michael Vaphiades, Magnetic resonance imaging in pseudotumor cerebri, Ophthalmology, 1998;105(9):1686−1693 [Fig. 2]. ISSN 0161-6420, https://doi.org/10.1016/S0161-6420(98)99039-X. (https://www.sciencedirect.com/science/article/pii/S016164209899039X).)

The Science Behind the Diagnosis

CLINICAL SYNDROME

An often-missed diagnosis, pseudotumor cerebri is a relatively common cause of headache. It has an incidence of 2.2 per 100,000 patients, approximately the same incidence as cluster headache. Primary pseudotumor cerebri is also known as idiopathic intracranial hypertension. If a clear etiology for the patient's intracranial hypertension is identified, some clinicians refer to this syndrome as secondary pseudotumor cerebri or secondary intracranial hypertension. Pseudotumor cerebri is seen most frequently in overweight women between the ages of 20 and 45 years. If epidemiologic studies look only at obese women, the incidence increases to approximately 20 cases per 100,000 patients. An increased incidence

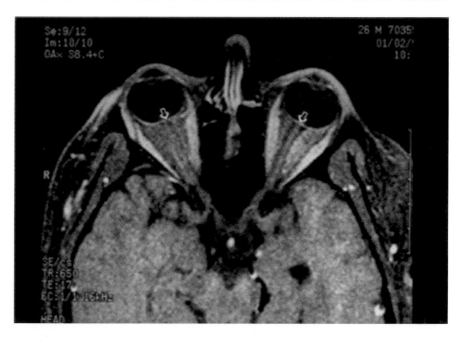

Fig. 9.3   Flattening of posterior sclera. T_1-weighted axial image with fat suppression shows bilateral flattening of the posterior sclera (arrows). (From Michael C Brodsky, Michael Vaphiades, Magnetic resonance imaging in pseudotumor cerebri, Ophthalmology, 1998;105(9):1686–1693 [Fig. 1]. ISSN 0161-6420, https://doi.org/10.1016/S0161-6420(98)99039-X. (https://www.sciencedirect.com/science/article/pii/S016164209899039X).)

of pseudotumor cerebri is also associated with pregnancy. The exact cause of pseudotumor cerebri has not been elucidated, but the common denominator appears to be a defect in the absorption of cerebrospinal fluid (CSF). Predisposing factors include ingestion of various medications, including tetracycline, vitamin A, corticosteroids, and nalidixic acid (Box 9.1). Other implicating factors include blood dyscrasias, anemias, endocrinopathies, and chronic respiratory insufficiency and anatomic abnormalities of the venous system and cerebrum that cause alterations in the flow of CSF. In many patients, however, the exact cause of pseudotumor cerebri remains unknown.

SIGNS AND SYMPTOMS

The diagnosis of pseudotumor cerebri is considered when a patient presents with the symptom triad of headache, visual changes, and papilledema, especially if the patient is female and obese (Fig. 9.5). More than 90% of patients suffering from pseudotumor cerebri present with the complaint of headache, are female, and have headaches that increase with the Valsalva maneuver.

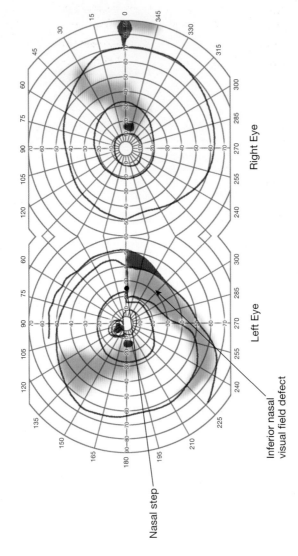

Left Eye

Right Eye

Nasal step

Inferior nasal
visual field defect

Fig. 9.4 The most common visual field defects associated with pseudotumor cerebri are an abnormally enlarged blind spot and a nasal step defect affecting the inferior quadrants of the visual field. (From Waldman S. *Atlas of Common Pain Syndromes*. ed. 4. Philadelphia: Elsevier; 2019 [Fig. 8.2]. 9780323547314.)

BOX 9.1 ■ Medications Reportedly Associated With Intracranial Hypertension

Vitamins
    Vitamin A
    Retinol
    Retinoids
Antibiotics
    Tetracycline and derivatives
    Nalidixic acid
    Nitrofurantoin
    Penicillin
Protein kinase C inhibitors
    Lithium carbonate
Histamine (H_2)-receptor antagonists
    Cimetidine
Steroids
    Corticosteroid withdrawal
    Levonorgestrel
    Danazol
    Leuprolide acetate
    Tamoxifen
    Growth hormone
    Oxytocin
    Anabolic steroids
Nonsteroidal antiinflammatory drugs
    Ketoprofen
    Indomethacin
    Rofecoxib
Antiarrhythmics
    Amiodarone
Anticonvulsants
    Phenytoin
Dopamine precursors
    Levodopa
    Carbidopa

Associated nonspecific central nervous system signs and symptoms, such as dizziness, visual disturbance including diplopia, tinnitus, photophobia, nausea and vomiting, and ocular pain can often obfuscate what should otherwise be a reasonably straightforward diagnosis, given that basically all patients suffering from pseudotumor cerebri (1) have papilledema on fundoscopic examination (see Fig. 9.1), (2) are female, and (3) are obese. The extent of papilledema varies from patient to patient and may be associated with subtle visual field defects, including an enlarged blind spot and inferior nasal visual field defects (see Fig. 9.4). If the condition is untreated, serious visual impairment may result (Fig. 9.6). Cranial nerve abnormalities may occur, with sixth cranial nerve palsy most common (Fig. 9.7).

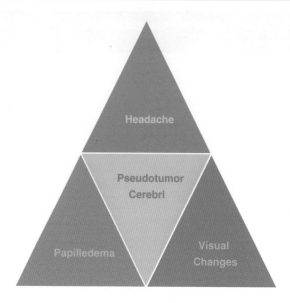

Fig. 9.5   The symptom triad of pseudotumor cerebri.

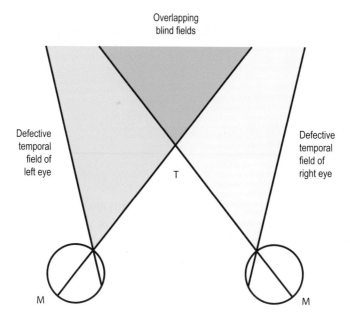

Fig. 9.6   Postfixation blindness associated with a complete bitemporal hemianopia in a patient with untreated pseudotumor cerebri. When the eyes converge and fix on a near target *(T)*, the blind temporal fields overlap behind it. Objects directly behind the target are invisible. *M*, Macula. (From Liu G, Volpe N, Galetta S. *Liu, Volpe, and Galetta's Neuro-Ophthalmology*. ed. 3. Philadelphia: Elsevier; 2019 [Fig. 7.10].)

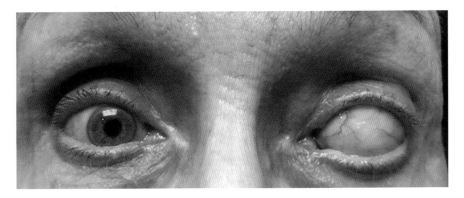

Fig. 9.7 Sixth cranial nerve palsy with complete abduction deficit. (From Gupta S, Ellis B, Hixenbaugh A, et al. Severe unilateral abducens nerve palsy from cavernous sinus carotid vascular ectasia. *Am J Ophthalmol Case Rep.* 2018;10:285−287 [Fig. 1]. ISSN 2451-9936, https://doi.org/10.1016/j.ajoc.2018. 04.006, http://www.sciencedirect.com/science/article/pii/S2451993617303298)

BOX 9.2 ■ Diagnostic Criteria for Primary Pseudotumor Cerebri (Idiopathic Intracranial Hypertension)

1. Signs and symptoms suggestive of increased intracranial pressure, including papilledema
2. Normal magnetic resonance imaging or computed tomography of the brain performed with and without contrast media reveals normal brain parenchyma with no evidence of hydrocephaly, masses, structural lesions, or meningeal enhancements
3. Increased cerebrospinal fluid (CSF) pressure documented by lumbar puncture
4. Normal CSF chemistry, cultures, and cytology

TESTING

By convention, the diagnosis of primary pseudotumor cerebri (idiopathic intracranial hypertension) is made when four criteria are identified: (1) signs and symptoms suggestive of increased intracranial pressure, including papilledema; (2) MRI or computed tomography (CT) of the brain reveals normal brain parenchyma with no evidence of hydrocephaly, masses, structural lesions, or meningeal enhancements; (3) increased CSF pressure documented by lumbar puncture; and (4) normal CSF chemistry, cultures, and cytology (Box 9.2). Urgent MRI and CT scanning of the brain with contrast media should be obtained on all patients suspected of having increased intracranial pressure to rule out intracranial mass, vascular abnormalities, and infection, among other disorders (Fig. 9.8). Once the absence of space-occupying lesions or dilated ventricles is confirmed on neuroimaging, it is safe to

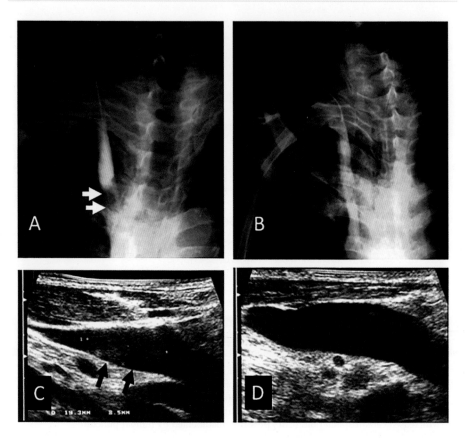

Fig. 9.8 (A) The pretherapeutic venogram of the right internal jugular vein (IJV), in frontal projection, shows the obstruction of the lower IJV. The arrows indicate the filling defect of the jugular vein thrombosis (JVT). (B) A posttherapeutic venogram obtained after anticoagulation therapy using warfarin shows the resolution and recanalization of the JVT. (C) A pretherapeutic ultrasonogram of the right internal jugular vein (IJV) shows the jugular vein thrombosis (JVT). The arrows indicate the thrombus in the right IJV. (D) A posttherapeutic ultrasonogram after the anticoagulation therapy using warfarin shows the resolution and recanalization of the JVT. (From Matsuda W, Noguchi S, Fujiyama F. Pseudotumor cerebri and lung cancer-associated jugular vein thrombosis: role of anatomical variations of torcular herophili. *Neurol Sci.* 2018;13:18—20 [Fig. 2]. ISSN 2405-6502, https://doi.org/10.1016/j.ensci. 2018.11.002, http://www.sciencedirect.com/science/article/pii/S2405650218300340)

proceed with lumbar puncture to measure CSF pressure and obtain fluid for chemistry, cultures, and cytology. Optical coherence tomography (OCT) may also be useful in monitoring the efficacy of interventions aimed at lowering CSF pressure. MRI findings that support the diagnosis of primary pseudotumor cerebri include (1) abnormalities of the sella turcica, including empty sella syndrome; (2) orbital abnormalities, including flattening of the posterior sclera of the globe and tortuosity of the optic nerves; and (3) bilateral optic disc protrusion (Fig. 9.9; see Figs. 9.2 and 9.3). CT scanning may

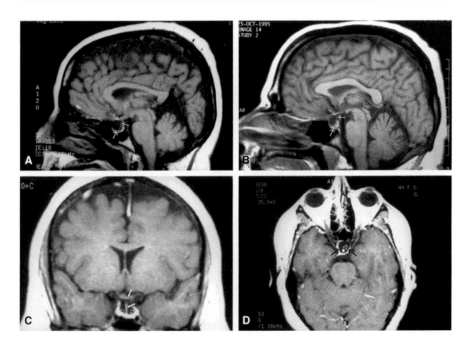

Fig. 9.9 Empty sella. A, T1-weighted sagittal magnetic resonance (MR) image shows small inferior crescent with concave upper surface corresponding to compressed pituitary gland (lower arrow). Note posterior displacement of the posterior infundibulum (middle arrow). Upper arrow denotes optic chiasm. Note abnormally prominent extraventricular subarachnoid space that appears hypointense and lies superior to the cerebral hemispheres. B, T1-weighted sagittal MR image shows a partially empty sella. Note concave upper pituitary surface and posterior displacement of the pituitary infundibulum (middle arrow). Upper arrow denotes optic chiasm, lower arrow denotes sellar floor. C, T1-weighted coronal MR image shows no visible pituitary gland within this portion of the sella. Open arrow denotes CSF-filled arachnocele, middle arrow denotes infundibulum, and upper arrow denotes optic chiasm. D, Enhanced T1-weighted axial MR image shows a hyperintense ring corresponding to the sella (open dark arrows), which contains a CSF-filled arachnocele. Intrasellar CSF appears as a discrete region of signal hypointensity surrounding a single focus of signal hyperintensity corresponding to a posteriorly displaced pituitary infundibulum (open white arrow). (From Michael C Brodsky, Michael Vaphiades, Magnetic resonance imaging in pseudotumor cerebri, *Ophthalmology*, 1998;105(9):1686–1693 [Fig. 1]. ISSN 0161-6420, Fig 6.)

reveal the unique finding of an increase in the area of the foramen ovale (Fig. 9.10).

DIFFERENTIAL DIAGNOSIS

If a specific cause is found for a patient's intracranial hypertension, it is by definition not idiopathic but a specific secondary type of intracranial hypertension (see Fig. 9.8). Causes of secondary pseudotumor cerebri or secondary intracranial hypertension that should be considered before diagnosing a patient with idiopathic intracranial hypertension are listed in Box 9.3. These include the various forms of intracranial hemorrhage, intracranial tumor,

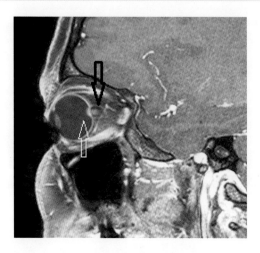

Fig. 9.10   T1 sagittal images with intravenous gadolinium reflects flattening of the posterior globe in a 22-year-old female with IIH and opening pressure of 42 cm H_2O and complaints of headache and tinnitus. There is obvious distension of the optic nerve sheath filled with CSF (black arrow) which results in optic disc being pushed into the globe (white arrow) resulting in the flattened globe posteriorly. There is also enhancement of the optic disc. IIH, idiopathic intracranial hypertension. (From Dirk Rehder, Idiopathic Intracranial Hypertension: Review of Clinical Syndrome, Imaging Findings, and Treatment, *Current Problems in Diagnostic Radiology*, 2020;49(3):205–214 [Fig. 6] ISSN 0363-0188, https://doi.org/10.1067/j.cpradiol.2019.02.012.)

cranial or cervical spine abnormalities such as Arnold-Chiari malformation, cerebral venous sinus thrombosis, abnormalities of the ventricular system, hepatic failure, and intracranial infections. A failure to diagnose a potentially treatable cause of intracranial hypertension may result in significant mortality and morbidity.

TREATMENT

A reasonable first step in the treatment of patients who exhibit all four criteria necessary for the diagnosis of pseudotumor cerebri is the initiation of oral acetazolamide. If poorly tolerated, the use of furosemide or chlorthalidone can be considered. A short course of systemic corticosteroids such as dexamethasone may also be used if the patient does not respond to diuretic therapy. The addition of weight-loss strategies in combination with the use of acetazolamide may hasten the resolution of the symptoms of pseudotumor cerebri. Early clinical reports suggest that octreotide, a synthetic somatostatin analogue, may be beneficial in the management of treatment-resistant pseudotumor cerebri. For resistant cases, neurosurgical interventions, including CSF shunt procedures, are a reasonable next step. If papilledema persists, decompression procedures on the optic nerve sheath have been advocated, as has the use of bariatric surgery.

BOX 9.3 ■ Common Causes of Secondary Intracranial Hypertension

Intracranial hemorrhage
   Intraventricular hemorrhage
   Subarachnoid hemorrhage
   Intraparenchymal hemorrhage
   Subdural hematoma
   Epidural hematoma
   Intracranial tumor
Primary brain tumors
   Meningiomas
   Pineal tumors
   Pituitary tumors
   Posterior fossa tumors
   Hamartomas
Cranial or cervical spine abnormalities
   Arnold-Chiari malformation
   Craniosynostosis
   Craniofacial dysostosis
Cerebral venous sinus thrombosis
Abnormalities of the ventricular system
   Aqueductal stenosis
   Dandy-Walker syndrome
Intracranial infections
   Meningitis
   Encephalitis
   Intracranial abscess
   Intracranial parasites
   Epidural abscess
Intracranial granulomas
   Eosinophilic granuloma
   Wegener granulomatosis
   Sarcoidosis
Lead poisoning

HIGH-YIELD TAKEAWAYS

- The patient is afebrile, making an acute infectious etiology unlikely.
- The patient is an obese female with a recent onset of holocranial headaches in the absence of antecedent trauma.
- The patient denies recent use of drugs associated with pseudotumor cerebri.
- MRI scanning demonstrates flattening of the posterior sclera, tortuous optic nerves, and bulging optic discs, which support the diagnosis of pseudotumor cerebri.
- The patient has an abnormal visual field test.

Suggested Readings

Beres SJ, Digre KB, Friedman DI, et al. Pseudotumor cerebri syndrome is the best term for this condition. *Pediatr Neurol.* 2018;87:9—10.

Eldweik L, McClelland C, Stein JD, et al. Association between cycline antibiotic and development of pseudotumor cerebri syndrome. *J Am Acad Dermatol.* 2019;81(2): 456—462.

Matsuda W, Noguchi S, Fujiyama F. Pseudotumor cerebri and lung cancer-associated jugular vein thrombosis: role of anatomical variations of torcular herophili. *Neurol Sci.* 2018;13:18—20.

Thurtell M. Update in the management of idiopathic intracranial hypertension. *Neurol Clin.* 2021;39(1):147—161.

Veiga-Canuto D, Carreres-Polo J. Role of imaging in pseudotumor cerebri syndrome. *Radiología* (English Edition). 2020;62(5):400—410.

Waldman SD. Pseudotumor cerebri. In: *Atlas of Common Pain Syndromes.* ed. 4. Philadelphia: Elsevier; 2019:29—31.

Waldman SD. Pseudotumor cerebri. In: *Pain Review.* ed. 2. Philadelphia: Saunders Elsevier; 2017:204—205.

Wall M. Update on idiopathic intracranial hypertension. *Neurol Clin.* 2017;35(1):45—57.

Shanice Williams

A 52-Year-Old Female With a Severe Headache and a Progressive Alteration of Consciousness

- Learn the common causes of intracranial hemorrhage.
- Develop an understanding of the clinical presentation of subarachnoid intracranial hemorrhage.
- Develop an understanding of how the physical findings can help the clinician determine the anatomic location of intracranial hemorrhage.
- Understand the difference between primary and secondary headaches.
- Develop an understanding of the role of computed tomography (CT) and CT angiography in the evaluation and treatment of subarachnoid intracranial hemorrhage.
- Develop an understanding of the treatment options for subarachnoid intracranial hemorrhage.
- Develop an understanding of the concept of "first or worst."
- Develop an understanding of the differential diagnosis of headache.
- Understand the risk factors for subarachnoid intracranial hemorrhage.
- Learn how to identify factors that cause concern.

Shanice Williams

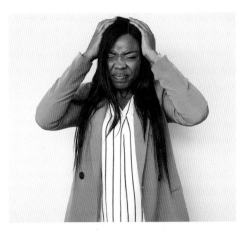

Shanice Williams is a 52-year-old book-keeper with the chief complaint of., "My head…my head…my head." Shanice was accompanied to the Emergency department (ED) by her husband, Bill, who provided the majority of the history, as Shanice was very somnolent. Her husband stated that Shanice was in their laundry room when he heard her cry out. He rushed to the laundry room, where he found Shanice sitting on the floor, leaning against the dryer, holding her head, and crying out in pain. He asked her what was wrong, and all she could say is what he thought was "my head…my head…my head." Bill grabbed Shanice's cell phone, which had fallen to the floor, and called 911. "Doctor, the ambulance arrived in about 3 minutes along with about 19 firefighters. The EMT said her blood pressure was off the charts, and he thought she was having a stroke. They loaded her into the ambulance, and I followed them to the hospital. At first, they told me to stay in the waiting room, but a couple of minutes later a nurse came out and asked me to come back so I could tell them what happened."

I was covering neurology and arrived at the bedside at about the same time as Bill, who quickly related what had happened. I explained to Bill that the ED physician believed that Shanice was suffering a stroke, so we needed to quickly determine what kind of stroke it was to best determine treatment options. I asked Bill when was the last time Shanice seemed normal, and he said, "Right when she walked into the laundry room, about 45 minutes ago, I think." Bill continued, "Doctor, do whatever you need to do to help Shanice! Should I call the kids?" I told him that while we were examining Shanice and getting a CT, he could go back out to the waiting area and I would come get him as soon as I had some answers. He could certainly call their kids and tell them for now that Shanice was safe and that we were getting the answers we needed to best treat her. "Bill, just a few quick yes-or-no questions: Is Shanice diabetic? Is she on blood thinners? Has she had a previous stroke? Does she have high blood pressure? Does she have atrial fibrillation or other types of abnormal heart beats? Any use of illicit drugs, cocaine, meth? Allergic to seafood or iodine?" Bill shook his head and answered no to all of these questions.

Shanice's vitals on admission to the ER were as follows: Her respirations were 20, her pulse oximetry was 98 on 2 L oxygen via nasal cannula, her pulse was 88 and regular, her blood pressure was 180/100, and she was afebrile. Her fingerstick blood sugar determination was 100. I performed a quick physical examination using the National Institute of Health Stroke Scale (NIHSS) to establish a neurologic baseline before we took Shanice to CT. Her level of consciousness revealed that she was somnolent but arousable with minor stimulation. Shanice was able to tell me how old she was, but she could not correctly identify what month it was. She was able to correctly respond to the commands "open and close your eyes" and "grip and release your hand." Shanice was able to follow my finger with her eyes on command. The visual threat maneuver suggested that Shanice had no visual loss. Mild facial asymmetry was noted on the left when Shanice was asked to "show me your teeth," "raise your eyebrows," and "close your eyes." She was able to maintain position of her arms bilaterally when the arms were extended with the palms down. There was also no lower extremity drift identified when each leg was extended 30 degrees. With encouragement, Shanice was able to "touch your finger to your nose" and "touch your heel to your shin." No sensory deficit was identified. I showed Shanice the NIHSS "Kitchen Disasters" picture and asked her what she saw (Fig. 10.1). Severe aphasia was identified, but when asked to point at was wrong in the picture, she

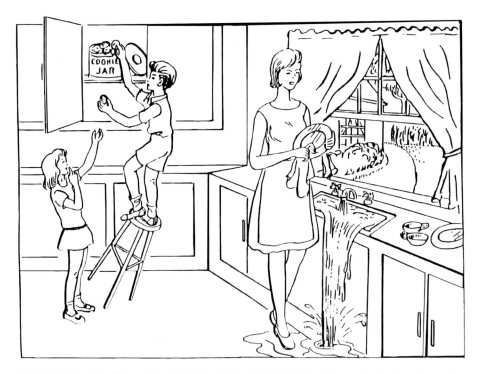

Fig. 10.1   National Institutes of Health Stroke Scale (NIHSS) "Kitchen Disasters" drawing. The patient is asked to tell the examiner what is displayed in the picture. (From https://www.ninds.nih.gov/sites/default/files/NIH_Stroke_Scale.pdf)

correctly identified the overflowing sink and the child falling off the stool. She was unable to name any of the items on the NIHSS "Name That Item" card but was able to correctly point to the items when I named them (Fig. 10.2). She was unable to read any of the sentences or say any of the words on the NIHSS sentence or word list. There was no evidence of visual or spatial inattention, and her fundoscopic examination was within normal limits. Her lungs were clear, her abdomen was soft without mass or organomegaly, and there was no obvious murmur or carotid bruit. At this point, the door-to-needle time was 22 minutes; we needed to get a move on to get her to CT.

It took less than 10 minutes to get a CT and I had my answer.

Key Clinical Points—What's Important and What's Not
THE HISTORY

- A history of sudden onset of severe "first or worst" headache with an alteration in consciousness
- Patient is afebrile
- No history of anticoagulants
- No history of previous stroke
- No history of cardiac arrythmia
- No history of diabetes
- No history of illicit drug use
- No allergy to seafood or iodine
- An inability to speak clearly

THE PHYSICAL EXAMINATION

- Patient is afebrile
- Patient is hypertensive
- Patient is somnolent but rousable with mild stimulation
- Patient is aphasic
- Patient has mild facial asymmetry
- Patient has no gross motor or sensory deficit
- Fundoscopic examination is normal

OTHER FINDINGS OF NOTE

- Normal cardiac examination
- Normal pulmonary examination
- Normal abdominal examination
- No carotid bruit

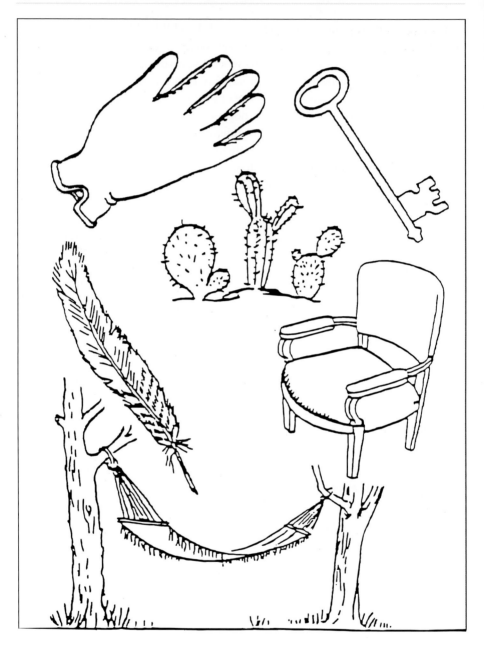

Fig. 10.2 National Institutes of Health Stroke Scale (NIHSS) "Name That Item" drawing. The examiner points to an item in the picture and asks the patient to tell the examiner what it is. (From https://www. ninds.nih.gov/sites/default/files/NIH_Stroke_Scale.pdf)

- Fingerstick blood glucose was 100
- Pulse oximetry on 2 L oxygen via nasal cannula was 98

 ## What Tests Would You Like to Order?

The following tests were ordered:
- CT scan of the brain with CT angiography
- Repeat blood glucose
- Troponin
- International normalized ratio (INR)
- Activated partial thromboplastin time (aPTT)
- Electrocardiogram (ECG)

TEST RESULTS

CT scan of the brain revealed a significant subarachnoid hemorrhage (SAH) (Fig. 10.3). CT angiography revealed a ruptured aneurysm of the right middle cerebral artery (Fig. 10.4). Repeat blood sugar was 97. Troponin, INR, and aPPT were all normal. Normal ECG.

 ## Clinical Correlation—Putting It All Together

What is the diagnosis?
Acute intracranial subarachnoid hemorrhage

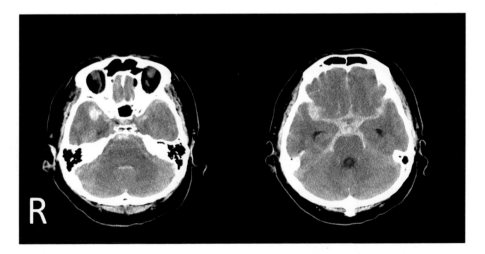

Fig. 10.3 Computed tomography scans obtained on admission show diffuse subarachnoid hemorrhage. (From Sato Y, Kojima T, Kawahara Y. Cognitive outcome in a patient with poor grade aneurysmal subarachnoid hemorrhage: focus on aphasia. *Interdisc Neurosurg*. 2019;18:100512 [Fig. 1]. ISSN 2214-7519, https://doi.org/10.1016/j.inat.2019.100513, http://www.sciencedirect.com/science/article/pii/S2214751919302002)

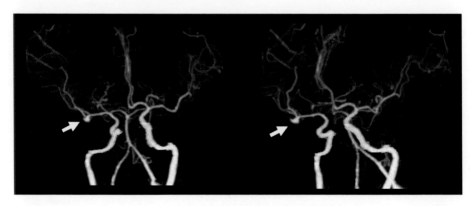

Fig. 10.4 Computed tomography angiography performed on admission suggests a ruptured aneurysm on the right middle cerebral artery *(arrowheads)*. (From Sato Y, Kojima T, Kawahara Y. Cognitive outcome in a patient with poor grade aneurysmal subarachnoid hemorrhage: focus on aphasia. *Interdisc Neurosurg.* 2019;18:100513 [Fig. 2]. ISSN 2214-7519, https://doi.org/10.1016/j.inat.2019.100513, http://www.sciencedirect.com/science/article/pii/S2214751919302002)

The Science Behind the Diagnosis

CLINICAL SYNDROME

Subarachnoid hemorrhage represents one of the most neurologically devastating forms of cerebrovascular accident (CVA). Fewer than 60% of patients suffering from the malady will recover cognitively and functionally to their premorbid state. From 65% to 70% of all SAH results from rupture of intracranial berry aneurysms. Arteriovenous malformations, neoplasm, and angiomas are responsible for most of the remainder (Fig. 10.5). Berry aneurysms are prone to rupture because of their lack of a fully developed muscular media and collagen-elastic layer. Systemic diseases associated with an increased incidence of berry aneurysm include Marfan syndrome, Ehlers-Danlos syndrome, sickle cell disease, coarctation of the aorta, alpha$_1$-antitrypsin deficiency, polycystic kidney disease, fibromuscular vascular dysplasia, and pseudoxanthoma elasticum (Box 10.1). Hypertension, alcohol and caffeine consumption, smoking, and cocaine use, which are modifiable risk factors, and cerebral atherosclerosis increase the risk of SAH. Black people are more than twice as likely to suffer SAH when compared with White people. Female patients may be affected slightly more often than male patients, and the mean age of patients suffering from SAH is 50 years. Even with modern treatment, the mortality associated with significant SAH is approximately 25%.

SIGNS AND SYMPTOMS

Massive SAH is often preceded by a warning in the form of what is known as a sentinel or thunderclap headache. This headache is thought to be the result of

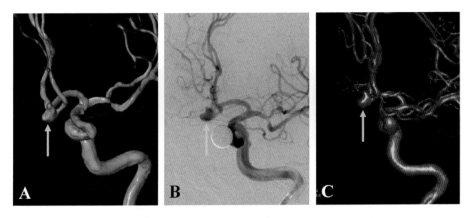

Fig. 10.5 Aneurysm in the left anterior communicating artery in a 61-year-old male patient with sub-arachnoid hemorrhage and a Glasgow Coma Scale score of 15. (A) Three-dimensional time-of-flight magnetic resonance angiography reveals an aneurysm *(arrow)* located at the left anterior communicating artery. (B) Digital subtraction angiography and (C) volume rendering digital subtraction angiograph demonstrate the aneurysm *(arrow)* located at the left anterior communicating artery. (From Yan R, Zhang B, Wang L, et al. A comparison of contrast-free MRA at 3.0 T in cases of intracranial aneurysms with or without subarachnoid hemorrhage. *Clin Imaging.* 2018;49:131−135 [Fig. 2]. ISSN 0899-7071, https://doi.org/10.1016/j.clinimag.2017.10.012, http://www.sciencedirect.com/science/article/pii/S0899707117302073)

BOX 10.1 ■ Systemic Diseases Associated With an Increased Incidence of Berry Aneurysm

Marfan syndrome
Ehlers-Danlos syndrome
Sickle cell disease
Polycystic kidneys
Coarctation of the aorta
Fibromuscular vascular dysplasia
Pseudoxanthoma elasticum

---

leakage from an aneurysm that is preparing to rupture. The sentinel headache is of sudden onset, with a temporal profile characterized by a rapid onset to peak in intensity. The sentinel headache may be associated with photophobia and nausea and vomiting. Of patients, 90% with intracranial SAH will experience a sentinel headache within 3 months of significant SAH.

Patients with significant SAH experience the sudden onset of severe headache, which the patient often describes as the worst headache ever experienced (Fig. 10.6). This headache is usually associated with nausea and vomiting, photophobia, vertigo, lethargy, confusion, nuchal rigidity, and neck and back pain (Box 10.2). The patient experiencing acute SAH appears acutely ill, and up to 50% will lose consciousness as the intracranial pressure rapidly rises in response

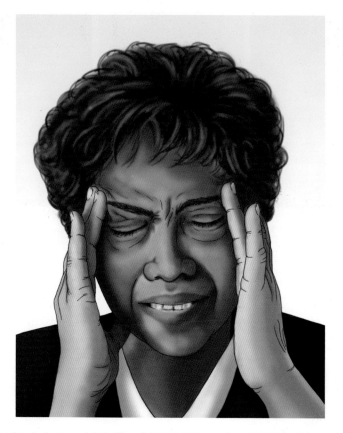

Fig. 10.6 The headache associated with subarachnoid hemorrhage is often described as the worst headache the patient has ever experienced. (From Waldman S. *Atlas of Common Pain Syndromes*. ed. 4. Philadelphia: Elsevier; 2019 [Fig. 9.2].)

BOX 10.2 ■ Symptoms Associated With Subarachnoid Hemorrhage

Severe headache
Nausea and vomiting
Photophobia
Vertigo
Lethargy
Confusion
Nuchal rigidity
Neck and back pain

---

to unabated hemorrhage. Cranial nerve palsy, especially of the abducens nerve, may also occur as a result of increased intracranial pressure. Focal neurologic signs, paresis, seizures, subretinal hemorrhages, and papilledema are often present on physical examination (Fig. 10.7).

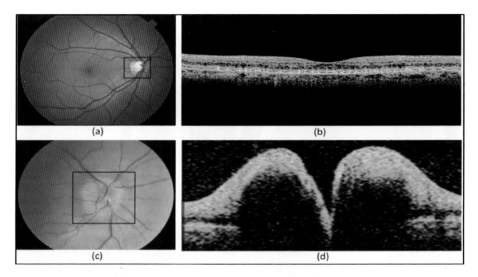

Fig. 10.7 Papilledema. (a) Normal fundus retinal image, (b) optical coherence tomograph and image of the head of the optic nerve (a). (c) Papilledema fundus retinal and (d) optical coherence tomograph and image of the head of the optic nerve (c). (From Akbar S, Akram MU, Sharif M, et al. Arteriovenous ratio and papilledema based hybrid decision support system for detection and grading of hypertensive retinopathy. *Comp Meth Progr Biomed.* 2018;154:123–141 [Fig. 6]. ISSN 0169-2607, https://doi.org/10.1016/j.cmpb.2017.11.014, http://www.sciencedirect.com/science/article/pii/S0169260717306661)

TESTING

Testing in patients suspected of suffering with SAH has two immediate goals: (1) to identify an occult intracranial pathologic process or other diseases that may mimic SAH and may be more amenable to treatment (see "Differential Diagnosis") and (2) to identify the presence of SAH. All patients with a recent onset of severe headache thought to be secondary to SAH should undergo emergency CT scanning of the brain (Fig. 10.8). Modern multidetector CT scanners have a diagnostic accuracy approaching 100% for SAH if CT angiography of the cerebral vessels is part of the scanning protocol (Fig. 10.9). Cerebral angiography may also be required if surgical intervention is being considered and the site of bleeding cannot be accurately identified. Because the MRI appearance of acute SAH evolves over time as the result of physical and chemical changes to the brain tissue in and around the hemorrhage, the sensitivity of MRI in acute SAH is less than that of CT angiography. Magnetic resonance imaging (MRI) of the brain and magnetic resonance angiography (MRA) may be useful if an aneurysm is not identified on CT studies and may be more accurate in the diagnosis of arteriovenous malformations (Fig. 10.10). Screening laboratory tests, including an erythrocyte sedimentation rate, complete blood count, coagulation studies, troponin, ECG, and automated blood chemistry, should be performed in patients suffering from SAH. Blood typing and crossmatching should be considered in

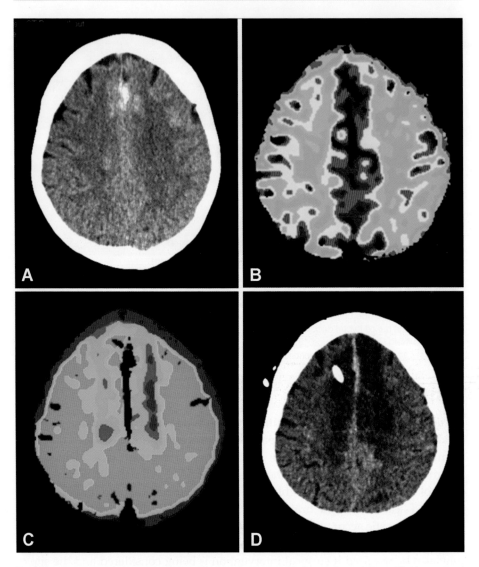

Fig 10.8 Computed tomography (CT) perfusion and the prediction of tissue infarct. (A) Noncontrast brain CT of a patient with severe anterior cerebral artery vasospasm showing subarachnoid hemorrhage in the anterior interhemispheric fissure secondary to a ruptured anterior communicating artery aneurysm. (B) There is no established infarct and normal cerebral blood volume on CT perfusion. (C) T_{max} maps show marked time delay to peak tissue perfusion and predict potential infarction in the anterior cerebral territory. (D) Brain CT 72 hours later confirms infarction in the predicted area with interval placement of a right frontal external ventricular drainage catheter. (From Li K, Barras CD, Chandra RV, et al. A review of the management of cerebral vasospasm after aneurysmal subarachnoid hemorrhage. *World Neurosurg.* 2019;126:513–527 [Fig. 1]. ISSN 1878-8750, https://doi.org/10.1016/j.wneu.2019.03.083, http://www.sciencedirect.com/science/article/pii/S187887501930751X)

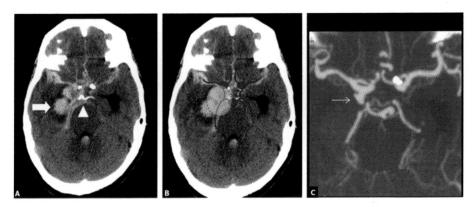

Fig. 10.9   Computed tomography (CT) and CT angiogram of the circle of Willis, performed in a patient with sudden-onset headaches, right third cranial nerve involvement, and abnormal consciousness. (A) Basal subarachnoid hemorrhage *(arrowhead)*, cisternal and medial cerebrotemporal hematoma *(arrow)*, ventricular hemorrhage visible in V4, and hydrocephalus with dilation of the left temporal horn. (B) Projection of the circle of Willis *(in red)*, and predominant site of blood *(orange circle)*, a localizing sign for investigation of the cause. (C) Confirmation of the suspected aneurysmal cause: ruptured aneurysm of the infundibulum of the right posterior cerebral artery *(arrow)*. (From Edjlali M, Rodriguez-Régent C, Hodel J, et al. Subarachnoid hemorrhage in ten questions. *Diagn Interv Imaging.* 2015;96[7–8]:657–666 [Fig. 3]. ISSN 2211-5684, https://doi.org/10.1016/j.diii.2015.06.003, http://www.sciencedirect.com/science/article/pii/S2211568415002107)

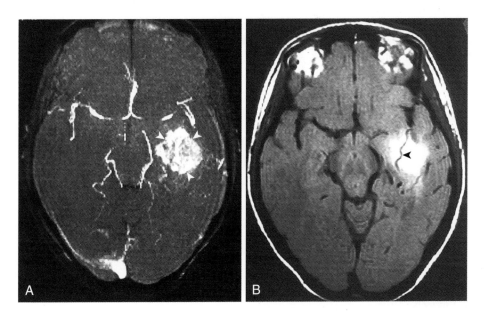

Fig. 10.10   Left temporal hemorrhage from an arteriovenous malformation. (A) On gradient-echo magnetic resonance imaging (MRI), the hematoma appears bright because of methemoglobin *(arrowheads)*, and no abnormal vessel is visualized. (B) On spin-echo MRI with flow presaturation below the section to be imaged, flow voids of abnormal vessels posterior to the hematoma and an abnormal vessel running through the hematoma *(arrowhead)* are visible. (From Mattle H, Edelman RR, Atkinson DJ. Zerebrale angiographie mittels kernspintomographie. *Schweiz Med Wochenschr.* 1992;122:323–333.)

any patient in whom surgery is being contemplated or who has preexisting anemia. Careful serial ophthalmologic examination and optical coherence tomography should be performed on all patients suffering from SAH to chart the course of papilledema (see Fig. 10.7).

Lumbar puncture may be useful in revealing blood in the spinal fluid, but its utility may be limited by the presence of increased intracranial pressure, which makes lumbar puncture too dangerous. Electrocardiographic abnormalities are common in patients suffering from SAH and are thought to result from abnormally high levels of circulating catecholamines and hypothalamic dysfunction.

DIFFERENTIAL DIAGNOSIS

For the most part, the differential diagnosis of SAH can be thought of as the diagnosis of the lesser of two evils because most of the diseases that mimic SAH are also associated with significant mortality and morbidity. Box 10.3 lists diseases that may be mistaken for SAH. Prominent among them are stroke, collagen vascular disease, infection, neoplasm, hypertensive crisis, spinal fluid leaks, and various, more benign causes of headache. With the advent of thrombolytic

---

BOX 10.3 ■ Diseases That May Mimic Subarachnoid Hemorrhage

Stroke (hemorrhagic)
Ischemic stroke
Neoplasm

Infection
Meningitis
Encephalitis
Abscess
Parasitic
Hypertensive encephalopathy
Loss of spinal fluid
Postdural puncture headache
Spontaneous spinal fluid leak
Collagen vascular disease
Lupus cerebritis
Vasculitis
Polymyositis
Bell palsy
Headache
Cluster headache
Thunderclap headache
Migraine
Seizures
Ice-pick headache
Sexual headache
Conversion reactions

therapy, the initial evaluation of a patient presenting with the acute symptoms that suggest stroke is focused on determining if the stroke is hemorrhagic or ischemic. Because the window of opportunity for the use of thrombolytic therapy for ischemic stroke is short, the door-to-needle time needs to be minimized. A standardized stroke evaluation protocol such as the NIHSS can facilitate timely evaluation of stoke victims and help optimize safe treatment.

TREATMENT

Medical management

The treatment of SAH begins with careful acute medical management, with an eye to minimizing the sequelae of both the cerebral insult and the morbidity associated with a severe illness. Bed rest with the head of bed elevated to 30 to 35 degrees to promote good venous drainage is a reasonable first step in the treatment of the patient suffering from SAH. Accurate intake and output determinations, as well as careful management of hypertension and hypotension, are also essential during the initial management of SAH, and invasive cardiovascular monitoring should be considered sooner rather than later in this setting. Pulse oximetry and end-tidal carbon dioxide monitoring should be initiated early in the course of treatment to identify respiratory insufficiency. Avoidance of overuse of opioids and sedatives is important to prevent hypoventilation with its attendant increase in intracranial pressure and cerebral ischemia. Seizure precautions and aggressive treatment of seizures are also required. Nimodipine, the calcium antagonist, is also recommended for prevention of delayed cerebral ischemia. Vomiting should be controlled to avoid the increase in intracranial pressure associated with the Valsalva maneuver. Prophylaxis of gastrointestinal bleeding, especially if steroids are used to treat increased intracranial pressure, and the use of pneumatic compression devices to avoid thrombophlebitis are also worth considering. If unconsciousness occurs, endotracheal intubation using techniques to avoid increases in intracranial pressure should be performed, and hyperventilation to decreased blood carbon dioxide levels should be considered.

Treatment of increased intracranial pressure with dexamethasone, the osmotic agent mannitol, and furosemide may be required. Calcium channel blockers and magnesium may be beneficial to reduce cerebrovascular spasm and decrease the zone of ischemia. Studies showed that statins may also be useful in this setting. Antifibrinolytics, such as epsilon-aminocaproic acid, may be useful to decrease the incidence of rebleeding in selected patients.

Surgical treatment

Surgical treatment of hydrocephalus with ventricular drainage may be required to treat highly elevated intracranial pressure, with the caveat that too rapid a

decrease in intracranial pressure in this setting may result in an increased incidence of rebleeding. Surgical treatment with clipping of the aneurysm or interventional radiologic endovascular occlusive coil treatment of continued
bleeding or rebleeding carries a high risk of morbidity and mortality, but it may
be necessary if more conservative treatments fail.

COMPLICATIONS AND PITFALLS

The identification of sentinel headache and subsequent aggressive treatment
before significant SAH occurs give the patient the best chance of a happy outcome. Treatment of significant SAH is difficult, and ultimately results are disappointing. Careful attention to initial and ongoing medical management,
with aggressive monitoring and treatment of associated hypertension and
hypotension and respiratory abnormalities, is crucial to prevent avoidable
complications.

Complications and pitfalls in the diagnosis and treatment of SAH generally
fall into three categories. The first category involves the failure to recognize a
sentinel hemorrhage and to evaluate and treat the patient before significant SAH
occurs. The second category involves misdiagnosis, which results in treatment
delays that ultimately cause an increase in mortality and morbidity. The third
category involves less than optimal medical management, which results in
avoidable mortality and morbidity. Examples are pulmonary embolus from
thrombophlebitis and aspiration pneumonia from failure to protect the patient's
airway.

HIGH-YIELD TAKEAWAYS

- The patient is afebrile, making an acute infectious etiology unlikely.
- The patient's CT and CT angiography is diagnostic for acute subarachnoid
  intracranial hemorrhage, which precludes the use of thrombolytic therapy.
- The major neurologic deficit identified at the time of initial evaluation is aphasia,
  which can result in significant disability for the patient.
- The lack of other systemic disease improves the recovery of patients with acute
  subarachnoid intracranial hemorrhage.

Suggested Readings

Abraham MK, Chang WW. Subarachnoid hemorrhage. *Emerg Med Clin North Am.*
    2016;34(4):901–916.
Edlow JA, Abraham MK. Neurologic emergencies—making the diagnosis and treating
    the life threats. *Emerg Med Clin North Am.* 2016;34(4):xvii–xviii.

Howard RS. The management of haemorrhagic stroke. *Anaesth Intens Care Med*. 2016;17(12): 596–601.

Malhotra A, Wu X, Gandhi D, et al. The patient with thunderclap headache. *Neuroimaging Clin North Am*. 2018;28(3):335–351.

Manhas A, Nimjee SM, Agrawal A, et al. Comprehensive overview of contemporary management strategies for cerebral aneurysms. *World Neurosurg*. 2015;84(4):1147–1160.

Perry JJ, Stiell IG, Sivilotti MA, et al. Clinical decision rules to rule out subarachnoid hemorrhage for acute headache. *JAMA*. 2013;310(12):1248–1255.

Waldman SD. Intracranial subarachnoid hemorrhage. In: *Atlas of Common Pain Syndromes*. ed. 4. Philadelphia: Elsevier; 2019:32–36.

Yan R, Zhang B, Wang L, et al. A comparison of contrast-free MRA at 3.0T in cases of intracranial aneurysms with or without subarachnoid hemorrhage. *Clin Imaging*. 2018;49:131–135.

Hattie Harrison

A 77-Year-Old Female With Headache and Jaw Pain

- Learn the common causes of headache.
- Learn the clinical presentation of temporal arteritis, including the unique symptom of jaw claudication.
- Learn how to use physical examination to identify physical findings associated with temporal arteritis.
- Learn to distinguish temporal arteritis from other pathologic processes that may mimic the disease.
- Learn the complications associated with temporal arteritis.
- Develop an understanding of the treatment options for temporal arteritis.

Hattie Harrison

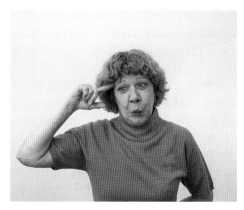

"I told Mom that she needed to see the doctor, but as usual, she wouldn't listen," complained Hattie's daughter, Betty. "She only wants to do what Hattie wants to do." I looked over at Hattie, who gave her daughter a dirty look and rolled her eyes. Hattie had been a patient of mine for several years and always came in for a flu shot, but otherwise I never saw her. Hattie was an original article: always cracking a joke and always ready to talk about Betty. Although she always had some criticism about Betty, it was obvious that she adored her. When she came in last fall for her flu shot, she brought me a copy of her Advanced Directives and Health Care Power of Attorney to put in her file. She became tearful, took my hand, and said, "Doctor, promise me that you will do whatever Betty tells you to do. I trust her to look after me like I looked after her. Nobody ever had a better daughter." I squeezed her hand and said, "I promise."

"Doctor, I told Betty I was fine! Just a little headache. You know, everybody gets a headache now and then. I am just fine," Hattie insisted. "I am a tough old bird." I took her hand and looked her straight in the eye and said, "Hattie, I know you are tough, but Betty is really worried about you. She says that you are having trouble chewing your food and you're losing weight. Let's see what we can do to get you back on your feet!" She gave her daughter a defiant look and said, "I told you I am fine. Go take care of people that actually have something wrong with them!"

Hattie told me that her headache pain began about 2 weeks ago. She said that it just gradually came on. At first it was just an ache, but lately it is more severe. She said, "Doctor, it's the craziest thing, but it hurts when I try to brush my hair." Hattie went on to say that over the last week she found it hard to get comfortable because her head hurt all the time. Tylenol and aspirin helped a little, but she finally agreed to come in because her jaw had started hurting whenever she tried to chew her food. "Doctor, it's kind of like a cramp in my jaw. If I try to keep chewing, the pain keeps getting stronger. If I rest for a minute, the cramping goes away, but if I try to chew again, the pain comes right back. It's very strange!"

I asked Hattie what made her pain worse and she said, "Chewing." I asked her what made the pain better, and she, without missing a beat, said, "Being left alone!" I laughed and asked if she had any problem going to the bathroom or was she losing any urine or feces or having any difficulty walking. Hattie shook her head adamantly from side to side. "Doctor, I can take care of myself." And looking straight at Betty, she said, "Nobody is going to put me in the old folks, home!" I reassured her that she wasn't going to the nursing home any time soon. I really didn't know what Betty had on her mind, though, because Betty could be as stubborn as her mother. I told Hattie I was going to take a look at her and see what we could do to get her better.

On physical examination, Hattie was afebrile. Her eye exam revealed dense bilateral cataracts. I really couldn't adequately visualize her optic discs. Her nose and throat examination, as well as her thyroid examination, were unremarkable. I asked Hattie if she was having any problem seeing or if anything had recently changed with her vision, and she snapped, "I can see better than you can!"

"Hattie, are you still driving?" I asked. Hattie glared at Betty and said, "Not since she took away my car keys!" "Mom," Betty said, "you know I will take you wherever you want to go." I made a note to refer Hattie to an ophthalmologist to look at her cataracts before she left the office.

Hattie's cardiopulmonary examination revealed a grade 2 mitral valve systolic murmur, which I had noted on previous visits. Her abdominal examination was benign, with no abnormal mass or organomegaly. There was a trace of peripheral edema. Hattie's radial pulses were 1 + bilaterally, but I was unable to identify any posterior tibial or dorsalis pedis pulses. What really concerned me was the finding of an inflamed, erythematous, thickened temporal artery on the left. The artery was easily visible and was so large that I could easily roll it between my fingers. A careful neurologic examination of the upper and lower extremities was unremarkable. No pathologic reflexes or clonus were identified.

Key Clinical Points—What's Important and What's Not
THE HISTORY

- History of jaw claudication associated with headache
- No significant history of previous headache
- Difficulty eating due to persistent jaw claudication
- Denies any recent decrease in visual acuity

THE PHYSICAL EXAMINATION

- Patient is afebrile
- Inflammation and thickening of the left temporal artery
- Dense cataract formation bilaterally
- No peripheral pulses in the lower extremities
- Normal neurologic examination

- No pathologic reflexes
- No clonus

OTHER FINDINGS OF NOTE

- Grade 2 mitral valve murmur

 ## What Tests Would You Like to Order?

- Urgent erythrocyte sedimentation rate (ESR)
- Urgent ultrasound and color Doppler image of the temporal arteries
- Urgent temporal artery biopsy
- Ultrasound of the aorta

TEST RESULTS

- ESR is 98.
- Ultrasound and color Doppler images of the temporal arteries reveal arterial luminal thickening and a positive halo sign, which is highly suggestive of temporal arteritis (Figs. 11.1, 11.2, and 11.3).

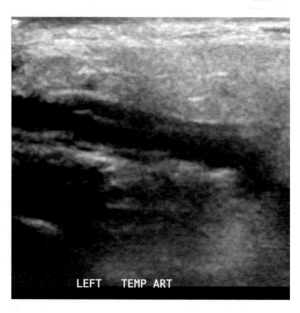

Fig. 11.1 Ultrasound of the left temporal artery with arterial wall thickening evident, consistent with temporal arteritis. (From Deyholos C, Sytek MC, Smith S, et al. Impact of temporal artery biopsy on clinical management of suspected giant cell arteritis. *Ann Vasc Surg.* 2020 [Fig. 1]. ISSN 0890-5096, https://doi.org/10.1016/j.avsg.2020.06.012, http://www.sciencedirect.com/science/article/pii/S0890509620305136)

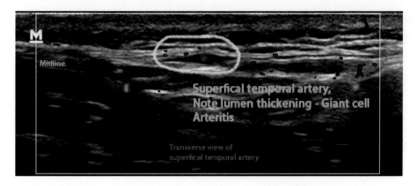

Fig. 11.2 Transverse color Doppler image of the temporal artery demonstrating arterial luminal thickening and a positive halo sign, which is highly suggestive of temporal arteritis.

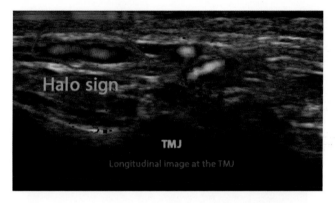

Fig. 11.3 Longitudinal color Doppler image in a patient with temporal arteritis demonstrating thickening of the wall of the temporal artery and a positive halo sign. Image is taken at the level just above the temporomandibular joint (TMJ).

- Temporal artery biopsy reveals lymphoplasmacytic infiltrate associated with internal elastic lamina and medial destruction with marked intimal hyperplasia with resultant luminal obstruction consistent with severe temporal arteritis (Fig. 11.4).
- Aortic ultrasound reveals thickening of the aortic wall with a large aortic dissection and associated false lumen and significant mural hematoma formation (Fig. 11.5).

Clinical Correlation—Putting It All Together

What is the diagnosis?
Temporal arteritis and aortic dissection

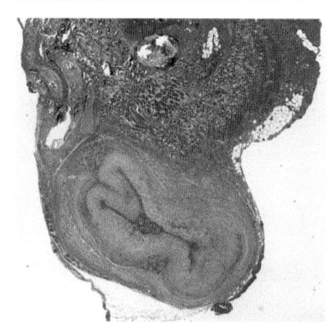

Fig. 11.4 Photomicrograph of temporal artery with lymphoplasmacytic infiltrate associated with internal elastic lamina and medial destruction with marked intimal hyperplasia with resultant luminal obstruction (Masson trichrome ×20). (From Pipinos II, Hopp R, Edwards WD, et al. Giant-cell temporal arteritis in a 17-year-old male. *J Vasc Surg.* 2006;43(5):1053–1055 [Fig. 2]. ISSN 0741-214, https://doi.org/10.1016/j.jvs.2005.12.043, http://www.sciencedirect.com/science/article/pii/S0741521406000061)

The Science Behind the Diagnosis

THE CLINICAL SYNDROME

As the name suggests, headache associated with temporal arteritis is located primarily in the temples, with secondary pain often located in the frontal and occipital regions (Fig. 11.6A). A disease of the sixth decade and beyond, temporal arteritis affects Whites almost exclusively, and there is a 3:1 female gender predominance. There is also a high correlation with smoking as well as a twofold increase in the incidence of aortic aneurysm. Temporal arteritis is also known as giant cell arteritis because of the finding of elastin-containing giant multinucleated cells that infiltrate arteries including the temporal, ophthalmic, and external carotid arteries (see Fig. 11.1). Approximately half of patients with temporal arteritis also have polymyalgia rheumatica. There is disagreement among clinicians as to whether temporal arteritis and polymyalgia rheumatica are different presentations of the same disease or entirely separate disease entities.

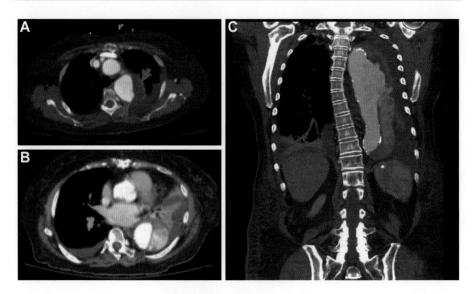

Fig. 11.5 Aortic dissection in a patient with temporal arteritis. Type B aortic dissection with interval expansion of the false lumen and increased aortic diameter of 6.3 × 6.9 cm. (A) Axial view with evidence of aortic ulcer *(red arrow)* and mural hematoma *(blue arrow)* at the proximal aorta. (B) Axial view with dissection flap seen within the aorta dividing native and false lumens and thickened aortic wall. (C) Coronal view of the aorta showing extensiveness of the false lumen and aneurysmal degeneration. (From Metias M, Kelian S, MacColl C, et al. Aortic dissection and accelerated aneurysmal degeneration in a patient with giant cell arteritis. *J Vasc Surg Case Innov Tech*. 2020 [Fig. 1]. ISSN 2468-4287, https://doi.org/ 10.1016/j.jvscit.2020.07.019, http://www.sciencedirect.com/science/article/pii/S2468428720301209)

SIGNS AND SYMPTOMS

Headache is seen in most patients with temporal arteritis. The headache is located in the temples and is usually continuous. The character of the headache pain associated with temporal arteritis is aching and has a mild to moderate level of intensity. A patient with temporal arteritis also may complain of soreness of the scalp, making the combing of hair or resting the head on a firm pillow extremely uncomfortable.

Although temporal headache is present in almost all patients with temporal arteritis, the finding of intermittent jaw claudication is pathognomonic for the disease (see Fig. 11.6B). In an elderly patient, jaw pain while chewing should be considered to be secondary to temporal arteritis until proved otherwise. In the presence of strong clinical suspicion that the patient has temporal arteritis, immediate treatment with corticosteroids is indicated (see "Treatment"). The reason immediate treatment is needed is the potential for sudden painless deterioration of vision in one eye secondary to ischemia of the optic nerve (Fig. 11.7).

In addition to the signs and symptoms mentioned previously, patients with temporal arteritis experience myalgia and morning stiffness. Muscle weakness

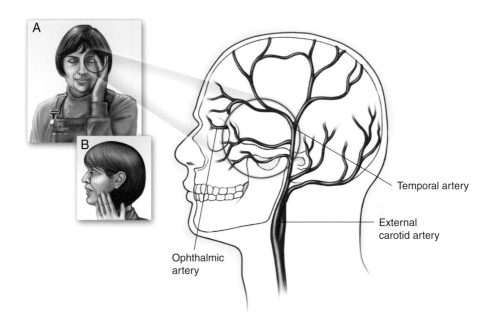

Fig. 11.6 (A) Temporal arteritis is a disease of the sixth decade that occurs almost exclusively in Whites, with a predilection of 3:1 for women. (B) The sine qua non of temporal arteritis is jaw claudication. (From Waldman S. *Atlas of Uncommon Pain Syndromes*. 4th ed. Philadelphia: Elsevier; 2020 [Fig. 12-1].)

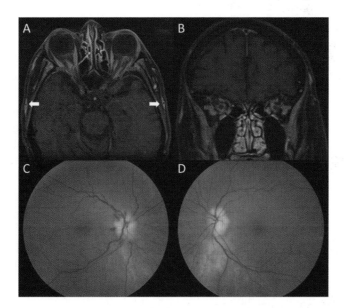

Fig. 11.7 Magnetic resonance imaging T1-weighted with contrast shows bilateral optic nerve sheath enlargement and enhancement on both axial (A) and coronal images (B) (*red arrows*). The axial images also show bilateral fusiform enlargement and enhancement of the temporal arteries (*white arrows*). Fundus photography demonstrates bilateral pallid disc edema (C, D) with a few peripapillary hemorrhages in the right eye (C). (From Chen J, Kardon R, Daley T, Longmuir R. Enhancement of the optic nerve sheath and temporal artieries from giant cell arteritis. *Can J Opthalmology, Correspondence*. 50(5): e96–e97, Fig. 1.)

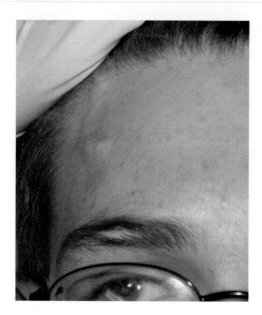

Fig. 11.8 Temporal arteritis. Note the dilated, tortuous temporal artery. (From Pipinos II, Hopp R, Edwards WD, et al. Giant-cell temporal arteritis in a 17-year-old male. *J Vasc Surg.* 2006;43(5):1053–1055 [Fig. 1]. ISSN 0741-5214, https://doi.org/10.1016/j.jvs.2005.12.043, http://www.sciencedirect.com/science/article/pii/S0741521406000061)

associated with inflammatory muscle disease and many other collagen vascular diseases is absent in temporal arteritis, unless the patient has been treated with prolonged doses of corticosteroids for other systemic disease, such as polymyalgia rheumatica. The patient also may experience nonspecific systemic symptoms, including malaise, weight loss, night sweats, and depression.

On physical examination, a swollen, indurated, nodular temporal artery is present (Fig. 11.8). Diminished pulses are often noted, as is tenderness to palpation. Scalp tenderness to palpation is often seen. Funduscopic examination may reveal a pale, chalky, edematous optic disc (Fig. 11.9). The patient with temporal arteritis often appears chronically ill, depressed, or both.

TESTING

ESR should be obtained in all patients suspected to have temporal arteritis. In temporal arteritis, the ESR is greater than 50 mm/hr in more than 90% of patients. Less than 2% of patients with biopsy-proved temporal arteritis have normal ESRs. Ideally, the blood for the ESR should be obtained before beginning corticosteroid therapy because the initial level of elevation of this test is useful not only to help diagnose the disease but also as a mechanism to establish the efficacy of therapy. The ESR is a nonspecific test, and other diseases that may

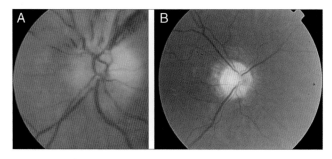

Fig. 11.9 Photographs of the optic disc in patients with giant-cell arteritis and visual loss due to anterior ischemic optic neuropathy, in the early acute phase (A) and after 3 months of prednisone therapy (B). (A) Optic disc oedema and a flame-shaped haemorrhage is shown. (B) Optic atrophy is shown. (Reprinted with permission from Elsevier (Carlo Salvarani FC, Hunder GG. Polymyalgia rheumatica and giant-cell arteritis, *Lancet*. 2008;372(9634):234–245, ISSN 0140-6736, Fig 2 https://doi.org/10.1016/S0140-6736(08)61077-6. (https://www.sciencedirect.com/science/article/pii/S0140673608610776))

manifest clinically in a manner similar to that of temporal arteritis, such as malignancy or infection, also may markedly elevate the ESR. Confirmation of the clinical diagnosis of temporal arteritis requires a temporal artery biopsy, although recent studies suggest that the use of ultrasound and color Doppler testing may mirror the sensitivity and specificity of temporal artery biopsy in the diagnosis of temporal arteritis (see Figs. 11.1, 11.2, and 11.3).

Given the simplicity and safety of temporal artery biopsy, it probably should be performed on all patients suspected of having temporal arteritis (Fig. 11.10). The presence of an inflammatory infiltrate with giant cells in the biopsied artery is characteristic of the disease (Fig. 11.11). Edema of the intima and disruption of the internal elastic lamina strengthen the diagnosis. A small percentage of patients with clinical signs and symptoms strongly suggestive of temporal arteritis who also exhibit a significantly elevated ESR have a negative temporal artery biopsy result. As mentioned, in the presence of a strong clinical impression that the patient has temporal arteritis, an immediate blood sample for ESR testing should be obtained and the patient started on corticosteroids. Complete blood cell count and automated chemistries, including thyroid testing, are indicated in all patients with suspected temporal arteritis to help rule out other systemic diseases that may mimic the clinical presentation of temporal arteritis.

If the diagnosis of temporal arteritis is in doubt, magnetic resonance imaging (MRI) of the brain provides the best information regarding the cranial vault and its contents. MRI is highly accurate and helps identify abnormalities that may put the patient at risk for neurologic disasters secondary to intracranial and brainstem pathologic conditions, including tumors and demyelinating

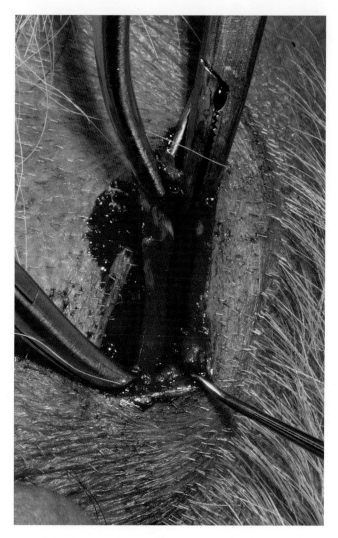

Fig. 11.10 Temporal artery biopsy. (From Markose G, Graham RM. Gillies temporal incision: an alternate approach to superficial temporal artery biopsy. *Br J Oral Maxillofac Surg.* 2017;55(7):719–721 [Fig. 2]. ISSN 0266-4356, https://doi.org/10.1016/j.bjoms.2017.05.002, http://www.sciencedirect.com/science/article/pii/S0266435617301535)

disease. More important, MRI helps identify bleeding associated with leaking intracranial aneurysms (Fig. 11.12). Magnetic resonance angiography (MRA) may be useful to help identify aneurysms responsible for neurologic symptoms. In patients who cannot undergo MRI, such as those with pacemakers, computed tomography (CT) and 18F-fluorodeoxyglucose positron emission tomography (PET)/CT are a reasonable second choice (Fig. 11.13).

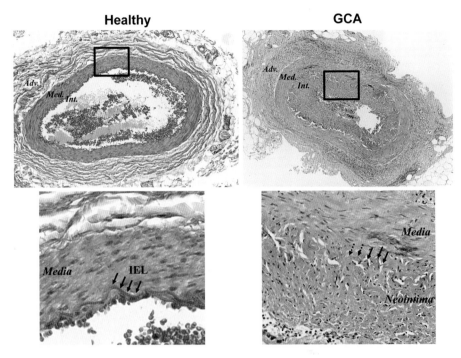

Fig. 11.11 Hematoxylin eosin safran staining of a healthy artery and of an artery affected by giant cell arteritis *(GCA)*. The healthy artery is characterized by a well-structured media and a thin intima separated by a preserved internal elastic lamina *(IEL)*. In the healthy artery, the artery wall is free of inflammatory cells, and its lumen is large. By contrast, many mononuclear inflammatory cells infiltrate the three layers of the artery affected by GCA (panarteritis). The media and the IEL are destroyed, thus allowing the migration and proliferation of vascular smooth muscle cells in the intima, leading to intimal hyperplasia and vascular occlusion. Magnification × 40. *Adv*, Adventitia; *int*, intima; *med*, media. (From Samson M, Corbera-Bellalta M, Audia S, et al. Recent advances in our understanding of giant cell arteritis pathogenesis. *Autoimmun Rev*. 2017;16(8):833–844 [Fig. 1]. ISSN 1568-9972, https://doi.org/10.1016/j.autrev.2017.05.014, http://www.sciencedirect.com/science/article/pii/S1568997217301386)

If intracranial hemorrhage is suspected, lumbar puncture should be performed, even if blood is not present on MRI or CT. Intraocular pressure should be measured if glaucoma is suspected.

DIFFERENTIAL DIAGNOSIS

Headache associated with temporal arteritis is a clinical diagnosis supported by a combination of clinical history, abnormal findings on physical examination of the temporal artery, normal radiography, MRI findings, an elevated ESR, and a positive temporal artery biopsy result. Pain syndromes that may mimic temporal arteritis include tension-type of headache, brain tumor, other forms of arteritis, trigeminal neuralgia involving the first division of the trigeminal nerve, demyelinating disease, migraine headache, cluster headache, and chronic paroxysmal

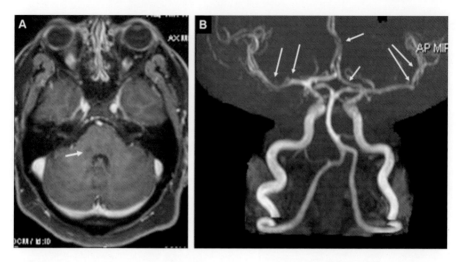

Fig. 11.12   Brain magnetic resonance imaging (MRI) and magnetic resonance angiography (MRA). A. Limited lesion in the right cerebellar tonsil (arrow) on MRI. B. Multifocal narrowing and irregularities within right anterior and distal middle cerebral artery branches, and milder irregularities of left anterior cerebral artery and bilateral posterior circulation on MRA. (McGeoch L, Sileckyc WB, Maherd J, Carettea S, Pagnouxa C. Temporal Arteritis in the young, *Joint Bone Spine*. 2013;80(3):324–327, Fig. 2.)

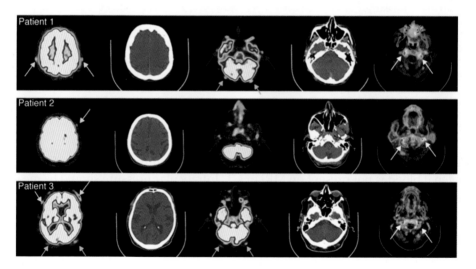

Fig. 11.13 ^{8}F-fluorodeoxyglucose (FDG) positron emission tomography/computed tomography (PET/CT) scan (axial slices), PET brain protocol—spectrum color scale, CT (same slice) and fusion PET/CT. High ^{18}F-FDG uptake is evident in temporal arteries *(red arrows)*, in their branches *(yellow arrows)*, occipital arteries *(green arrows)*, and vertebral arteries *(white arrows)*. (From Rehak Z, Vasina J, Ptacek J, et al. PET/CT in giant cell arteritis: high 18F-FDG uptake in the temporal, occipital and vertebral arteries. *Revista Española de Medicina Nuclear e Imagen Molecular (English Edition)*. 2016;35(6):398–401 [Fig. 2]. ISSN 2253-8089, https://doi.org/10.1016/j.remnie.2016.03.008, http://www.sciencedirect.com/science/article/pii/S2253808916300702)

TABLE 11.1 ■ Clinical Syndromes That Can Mimic Temporal Arteritis

- Acute herpes zoster
- Acute angle-closure glaucoma
- Iritis
- Uveitis
- Postherpetic neuralgia
- Cluster headache
- Migraine headache
- Ischemic optic neuropathy
- Ramsay-Hunt syndrome
- Polymyalgia rheumatica
- Wegener granulomatosis
- Collagen vascular disease
- Retinal artery occlusion
- Retinal vein occlusion
- Rheumatoid arthritis
- Subarachnoid hemorrage
- Transient ischemic attack

hemicrania (Table 11.1). Trigeminal neuralgia involving the first division of the trigeminal nerve is uncommon and is characterized by trigger areas and ticlike movements. Demyelinating disease is generally associated with other neurologic findings, including optic neuritis and other motor and sensory abnormalities. The pain of chronic paroxysmal hemicrania and cluster headache is associated with redness and watering of the ipsilateral eye, nasal congestion, and rhinorrhea during the headache. These findings are absent in all types of sexual headache. Migraine headache may or may not be associated with painless neurologic findings known as aura, but the patient almost always reports some systemic symptoms, such as nausea or photophobia, not typically associated with the headache of temporal arteritis.

TREATMENT

The mainstay of treatment for temporal arteritis and its associated headaches and other systemic symptoms is the immediate use of corticosteroids. If visual symptoms are present, an initial dose of 80 mg of prednisone is indicated. This dose should be continued until the symptoms of temporal arteritis have completely abated. At this point, the dose may be decreased by 5 mg/wk as long as the symptoms remain quiescent and the ESR does not increase. Cytoprotection of the stomach mucosa should be considered because ulceration and gastrointestinal bleeding are possible. If the patient cannot tolerate corticosteroids, or the maintenance dose of steroids remains so high as to produce adverse effects, the interleukin-6 (IL-6) receptor blocker tocilizumab is a reasonable next choice. Other immunosuppressive agents such as azathioprine or methotrexate are alternative options as steroid-sparing agents later in the course of the disease. Treatment of aortic disease will decrease the life-threatening complications associated with giant cell arteritis—induced abnormalities of the aorta (Fig. 11.14).

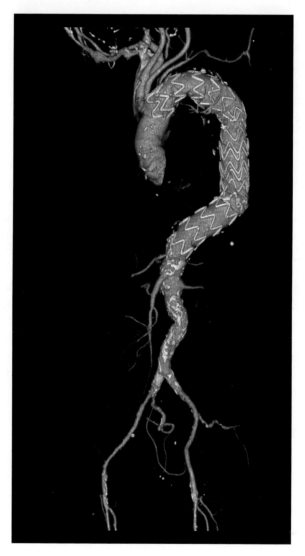

Fig. 11.14 Three-dimensional rendition of the aorta with endovascular repair of the aortic dissection and aneurysm in the descending aorta on postoperative day 1. The proximal fixation of the stent graft is at the origin of the innominate artery, and distal fixation is at the level of the celiac axis. (From Metias M, Kelian S, MacColl C, et al. Aortic dissection and accelerated aneurysmal degeneration in a patient with giant cell arteritis. *J Vasc Surg Case Innov Tech.* 2020 [Fig. 3]. ISSN 2468-4287, https://doi.org/10.1016/j.jvscit.2020.07.019, http://www.sciencedirect.com/science/article/pii/S2468428720301209)

COMPLICATIONS AND PITFALLS

The diagnosis of headache associated with temporal arteritis is made by obtaining a thorough, targeted headache history. As mentioned, jaw claudication is pathognomonic for temporal arteritis, and its presence should be sought in all elderly patients presenting with headache. Failure to recognize, diagnose, and treat temporal arteritis promptly may result in the permanent loss of vision.

Failure to diagnose the headache associated with temporal arteritis correctly may put the patient at risk if an intracranial pathologic condition or demyelinating disease (which may mimic the clinical presentation of temporal arteritis) is overlooked. MRI of the brain is indicated in all patients thought to have headaches associated with temporal arteritis. Failure to diagnose glaucoma, which also may cause intermittent ocular pain and mimic the clinical presentation of temporal arteritis, may result in permanent loss of sight.

HIGH-YIELD TAKEAWAYS

- Jaw claudication is pathognomonic for temporal arteritis.
- Temporal arteritis is a medical emergency that requires urgent and aggressive treatment to prevent visual loss and other complications of vasculitis.
- The patient is afebrile, making an acute infectious etiology (e.g., intracranial abscess or meningitis) unlikely.
- The patient's symptomatology is the result of inflammation of the arteritis.
- Treat with high-dose prednisone as soon as the diagnosis of temporal arteritis is suspected, even before temporal artery ultrasound and biopsy have been performed.
- Aortic complications can occur even after temporal arteritis treatment has been started.

Suggested Readings

Coronel L, Rodríguez-Pardo J, Monjo I, et al. Prevalence and significance of ischemic cerebrovascular events in giant cell arteritis. *Medicina Clín.* 2020;256−261.

Deshayes S, de Boysson H, Dumont A, et al. An overview of the perspectives on experimental models and new therapeutic targets in giant cell arteritis. *Autoimmun Rev.* 2020;19(10):102636.

Koster MJ, Yeruva K, Crowson CS, et al. Giant cell arteritis and its mimics: a comparison of three patient cohorts. *Sem Arthr Rheum.* 2020;50(5):923−929.

Nielsen BD, Gormsen LC. 18F-fluorodeoxyglucose PET/computed tomography in the diagnosis and monitoring of giant cell arteritis. *PET Clin.* 2020;15(2):135−145.

Rinagel M, Chatelus E, Jousse-Joulin S, et al. Diagnostic performance of temporal artery ultrasound for the diagnosis of giant cell arteritis: a systematic review and meta-analysis of the literature. *Autoimmun Rev.* 2019;18(1):56–61.

Waldman SD. Polymyalgia rheumatica. In: *Pain Review.* 2nd ed. Philadelphia: Saunders; 2017:324–326.

Waldman SD. Temporal arteritis. In: *Pain Review.* 2nd ed. Philadelphia: Saunders; 2017:199–200.

Lynn Sparks

A 26-Year-Old Sales Associate With Sharp, Stabbing Pain With Swallowing

Lynn Sparks

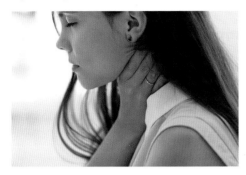

"It hurts every time I swallow and every time I turn my head to the left," complained Lynn Sparks. Lynn had been my patient for a couple of years. She was a senior sales associate at our local Dillard's. I had seen Lynn before for an uncomplicated urinary tract infection. Lynn had called the office earlier in the week and asked if we could work her in because she thought she had an ear infection. She recognized that she didn't have the usual fever that goes along with ear infections but decided to keep the appointment because her pain was not getting any better. I asked Lynn if she had experienced any fever or chills, and she shook her head no.

I asked Lynn if she had ever had anything like this before, and she shook her head no. "So, no fever or chills. Did you choke on anything or accidently swallow a bone?" Again, she shook her head no. l suggested that we look her over to figure out what was wrong, so we could make it better.

I asked Lynn to point with one finger where it hurts the most. Lynn pointed to her right anterior neck. "It starts right here, and when I swallow or turn my head to the left, I get this electric shock up into my jaw and ear."

"Is there any numbness?" I asked. Lynn replied that she hadn't noticed any. "You know, Doctor, this pain is making it hard to get any rest because if I swallow or roll over at night, I get the pain."

"Are you having any visual problems, or is there anything else that I need to know about?" I asked. Lynn replied, "Nothing else. Other than this pain, I feel fine." Lynn's last menstrual period was 1 week ago.

On physical examination, Lynn was afebrile and her respirations were 16. Her pulse was 74 and regular with a blood pressure of 110/68. Palpation of her cranium revealed no mass or other abnormality. Her fundoscopic examination was normal. A careful examination of the ears bilaterally were completely normal. Examination of her throat was normal, with evidence of a previous tonsillectomy. Her dentition was normal, with no impacted wisdom teeth. Her cardiopulmonary examination was normal. Her abdominal examination revealed no abnormal mass or organomegaly. There was no costovertebral angle (CVA) tenderness. There was no peripheral edema. Palpation over the right anterolateral neck at the level of the cricothyroid cartilage elicited a shocklike pain that radiated from the point of palpation to her contralateral ear and jaw. When I had Lynn turn her head to the left as far as she could, she again experienced the pain: nuchal ridge to the top of her head on the left. Her neurologic examination was otherwise within normal limits. There were no pathologic reflexes.

Key Clinical Points—What's Important and What's Not

THE HISTORY

- History of recent onset of right-sided anterolateral neck pain that was triggered with swallowing and turning the head to the left
- Swallowing and turning the head to the left also elicited an electric shocklike pain that radiated into the right ear and jaw
- Patient denies fever or chills
- Patient denies choking on food or accidently swallowing a bone
- No history of previous headache or facial pain

THE PHYSICAL EXAMINATION

- Patient is afebrile
- Pain elicited with palpation of the right anterolateral neck
- Pain elicited with swallowing and the turning of the head to the left
- Normal fundoscopic examination
- Normal neurologic examination, upper extremity motor and sensory examination
- No pathologic reflexes

OTHER FINDINGS OF NOTE

- Normal ears, nose, throat (ENT) examination
- Normal cardiovascular examination
- Normal pulmonary examination
- Normal abdominal examination
- No peripheral edema

What Tests Would You Like to Order?

The following tests were ordered:
- Radiographs of the neck
- Computed tomography (CT) of the neck

TEST RESULTS

Lateral cervical radiographs of the neck revealed an elongated styloid process (Fig. 12.1). The three-dimensional CT reconstruction of the neck revealed an elongated styloid process consistent with Eagle syndrome on the right (Fig. 12.2).

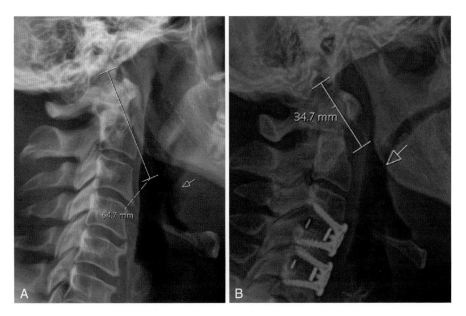

Fig. 12.1 Lateral cervical radiographs of two subjects with elongated styloid processes. (A) A styloid length of 64.7 mm. The arrow points to the second elongated styloid. (B) A styloid length of 34.7 mm. The arrow points to calcifications extending down from the styloid toward the hyoid bone. (From Westbrook AM, Kabbaz VJ, Showalter CR. Eagle's syndrome, elongated styloid process and new evidence for pre-manipulative precautions for potential cervical arterial dysfunction. *Musculoskel Sci Pract*. 2020;102219 [Fig. 6]. ISSN 2468-7812, https://doi.org/10.1016/j.msksp.2020.102219, http://www.sciencedirect.com/science/article/pii/S2468781220301399)

Clinical Correlation—Putting It All Together

What is the diagnosis?
Eagle syndrome

The Science Behind the Diagnosis

CLINICAL SYNDROME

An uncommon cause of facial pain, Eagle syndrome (also known as stylohyoid syndrome) is caused by pressure on the internal carotid artery and surrounding structures, including branches of the glossopharyngeal nerve, by an abnormally elongated styloid process, a calcified stylohyoid ligament, or both. The pain of Eagle syndrome is sharp and stabbing and occurs with movement of the mandible, swallowing, or turning of the neck (Fig. 12.3). The pain starts below the angle of the mandible and radiates into the tonsillar fossa, temporomandibular joint, and base of the tongue. A trigger point may be present in the tonsillar fossa.

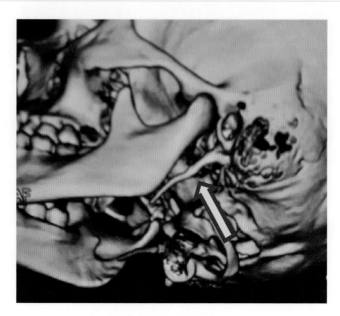

Fig. 12.2 Three-dimensional computed tomography radiograph showing an elongated styloid process in a patient with Eagle syndrome. (From Mahmoud NR, Ashour EM. Cervico-facial pain associated with Eagle's syndrome misdiagnosed as cranio-mandibular disorders. A retrospective study. *J Cranio-Maxillofac Surg*. 2020;48(10):1009–1017 [Fig. 4]. ISSN 1010-5182, https://doi.org/10.1016/j.jcms.2020.07.016, http://www.sciencedirect.com/science/article/pii/S1010518220301815)

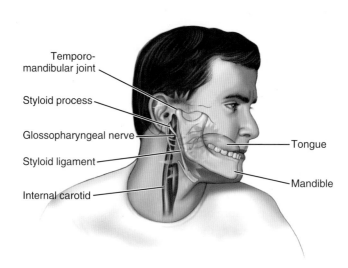

Fig. 12.3 The pain of Eagle syndrome is triggered by swallowing, movement of the mandible, or turning of the neck. (From Waldman S. *Atlas of Uncommon Pain Syndromes*. 4th ed. Philadelphia: Elsevier; 2020 [Fig. 15-1].)

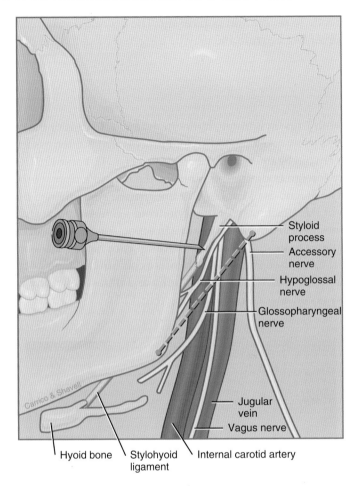

Styloid
process

Accessory
nerve

Hypoglossal
nerve

Glossopharyngeal
nerve

Jugular
vein

Vagus nerve

Hyoid bone   Stylohyoid   Internal carotid artery
                       ligament

Fig. 12.4   Injection technique for the treatment of Eagle syndrome. (From Waldman S. *Atlas of Pain Management Injection Techniques*. 4th ed. St. Louis: Elsevier; 2017 [Fig. 10-4]. 978-0-323-41415-9.)

Injection of the attachment of the stylohyoid ligament to the styloid process with local anesthetic and steroid serves as a diagnostic maneuver and a therapeutic maneuver (Fig. 12.4).

SIGNS AND SYMPTOMS

Eagle syndrome is most often a diagnosis of exclusion. Patients suffering from Eagle syndrome present with a history of sudden, sharp neuritic pain that begins below the angle of the mandible and radiates into the tonsillar fossa, temporomandibular joint, and base of the tongue. The pain is triggered by swallowing, movement of the mandible, or turning of the neck (see Fig. 12.3). The intensity of pain is moderate to severe and unpleasant. The neurologic examination is normal. The pain of Eagle syndrome may be triggered by palpation of the tonsillar fossa.

TESTING

In patients with Eagle syndrome, radiographs and CT scans of the region of the styloid process show an elongated styloid process that is often associated with a calcified stylohyoid ligament (Fig. 12.5; see also Figs. 12.1 and 12.2). CT may also help identify foreign bodies responsible for the patient's pain symptomatology (Fig. 12.6). The diagnosis of Eagle syndrome may be strengthened by a diagnostic injection of the attachment of the stylohyoid ligament to the styloid process with local anesthetic. Pain relief after this injection suggests a local cause for the pain rather than a more distant cause, such as glossopharyngeal neuralgia or retropharyngeal tumor (see Fig. 12.4). If there is a concern that injury of the adjacent carotid artery has occurred, CT angiography and ultrasonography will be helpful in identify occult aneurysm or bleeding (Fig. 12.7).

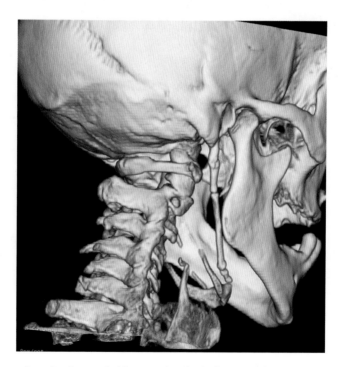

Fig. 12.5 Three-dimensional computed tomography clearly shows a stylohyoid ligament ossified from the base of the skull all the way into the anterolateral hyoid bone with a stylohyoid joint. (From Ata-Ali J, Ata-Ali F, Melo M, et al. Eagle syndrome compared with stylohyoid syndrome: complete ossification of the stylohyoid ligament and joint. *Br J Oral Maxillofac Surg.* 2017;55(2):218–219 [Fig. 1].)

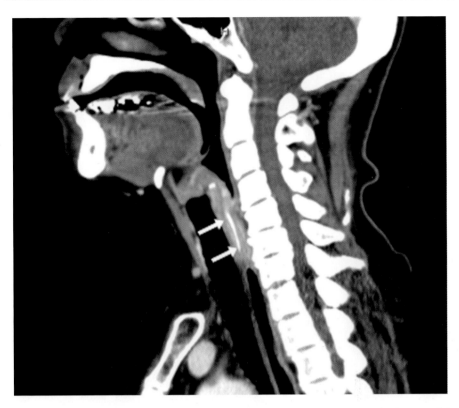

Fig. 12.6 Sagittal CT scans obtained with soft tissue technique. A fish bone located submucosally in the upper esophagus (arrow). (From Shintaro Baba, Katsumi Takizawa, Chikako Yamada, Hiroko Monobe, A submucosal esophageal fish bone foreign body surgically removed using intraoperative ultrasonography, *Am J Otolaryngol*, 2014;35(2):268–270, Fig. 1, ISSN 0196-0709, https://doi.org/10.1016/j.amjoto.2013.10.006 (https://www.sciencedirect.com/science/article/pii/S0196070913002470))

DIFFERENTIAL DIAGNOSIS

Eagle syndrome can be distinguished from glossopharyngeal neuralgia because the pain of glossopharyngeal neuralgia is characterized by paroxysms of shocklike pain in a manner analogous to trigeminal neuralgia, rather than the sharp, shooting pain on movement that is associated with Eagle syndrome. Because glossopharyngeal neuralgia may be associated with serious cardiac bradyarrhythmias and syncope, the clinician must distinguish the two syndromes.

The clinician should always evaluate a patient with pain in this anatomic region for occult malignancy. Tumors of the larynx, hypopharynx, and anterior triangle of the neck may manifest with clinical symptoms identical to those of Eagle syndrome. Because of the low incidence of Eagle syndrome

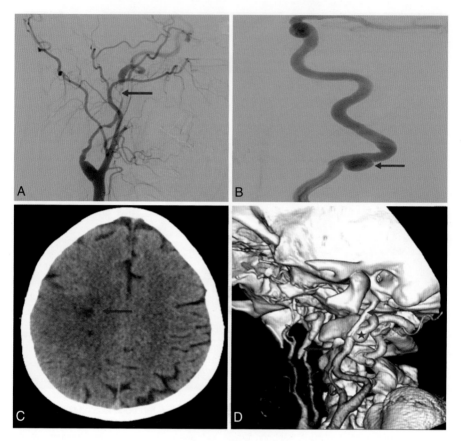

Fig. 12.7 (A) Right internal carotid dissection *(red arrow)* and (B) left internal carotid pseudoaneurysm *(red arrow)* confirmed with angiography. (C) Axial nonenhanced brain computed tomography (CT) showing several right frontal sequel ischemic lesions with sulci effacement. (D) Three-dimensional reconstruction CT with both elongated styloid processes *(red arrows)* and left pseudoaneurysm *(red star)*. (From Brassart N, Deforche M, Goutte A, et al. A rare vascular complication of Eagle syndrome highlight by CTA with neck flexion. *Radiol Case Rep.* 2020;15(8):1408–1412 [Fig. 1]. ISSN 1930-0433, https://doi.org/10.1016/j.radcr. 2020.05.052, http://www.sciencedirect.com/science/article/pii/S1930043320302296)

relative to pain secondary to malignancy and other causes of pain in this anatomic region, Eagle syndrome must be considered a diagnosis of exclusion (Table 12.1).

TREATMENT

Many patients with Eagle syndrome respond to a series of therapeutic injections of the attachment of the stylohyoid ligament to the styloid process with local anesthetic and steroid. To perform this procedure, an imaginary line is visualized running from the mastoid process to the angle of the mandible

TABLE 12.1 ■ **Differential Diagnoses for Patients With Eagle Syndrome**

Foreign body
Carotodynia
Cervical radiculopathy
Rheumatoid arthritis involving the upper cervical facet joints
Osteoarthritis involving the upper cervical facet joints
Temporomandibular joint disorders
Arnold-Chiari malformation
Acceleration-deceleration injuries
Iatrogenic damage to local nerves
Atlantoaxial subluxation
Atlantoaxial lateral masses
Glossopharyngeal neuralgia
Ontogenic disease
Piriformis fossa tumor
Obstruction of the tear duct
Obstruction of the eustachian tube
Ramsay Hunt syndrome
Acute herpes zoster
Zoster sine herpete
Postherpetic neuralgia
Sluder neuralgia
Carotid artery aneurysm
Angina
Trigeminal autonomic cephalgias
Neurofibromatosis type 1
Paget disease
Giant cell arteritis
Hemicrania continua

(see Fig. 12.4). The styloid process should lie just below the midpoint of this line. The skin is prepared with antiseptic solution. A 22-gauge, 1.5-inch needle attached to a 14-mL syringe is advanced at this midpoint location in a plane perpendicular to the skin. The styloid process should be encountered within 3 cm. After contact is made, the needle is withdrawn slightly out of the periosteum or substance of the calcified ligament. After careful aspiration reveals no blood or cerebrospinal fluid, 5 mL of 0.5% preservative-free lidocaine combined with 80 mg of methylprednisolone is injected in incremental doses. Subsequent daily nerve blocks are performed in a similar manner, substituting 40 mg of methylprednisolone for the initial 80-mg dose. Ultrasound guidance may increase the accuracy of needle placement and decrease the incidence of needle-induced complications (Fig. 12.8). Color Doppler imaging will add in the identification for the carotid artery and internal jugular vein (Fig. 12.9).

The sharp, shooting pain associated with Eagle syndrome also may be treated with gabapentin. Gabapentin is started at a single nighttime dose of 300 mg and titrated by 300-mg increments every 2 days in divided doses until pain relief is

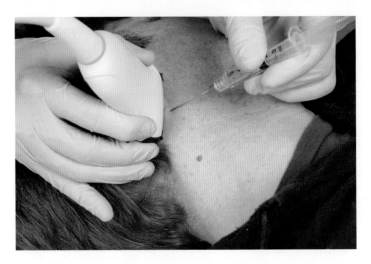

Fig. 12.8   Out-of-plane approach for ultrasound-guided injection of the styloid process.

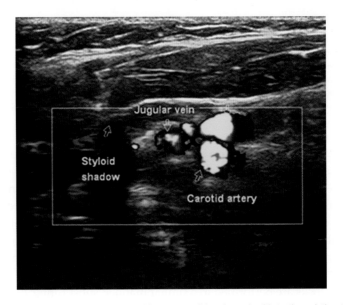

Fig. 12.9   Color Doppler image of the carotid artery and jugular vein. Note the relationship of these structures to the styloid process.

achieved or a total daily dose of 3600 mg is reached. Alternatively, carbamaze-pine, pregabalin, or phenytoin may be considered. In rare cases, surgical removal of the elongated styloid process may be necessary to provide

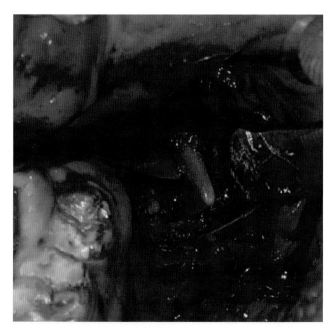

Fig. 12.10 Intraoral intraoperative photograph of an excision of the styloid process in a patient suffering from Eagle syndrome that failed to respond to medication management and injections with local anethestic and steroids. Note the elongated styloid process. (From Mahmoud NR, Ashour EM. Cervico-facial pain associated with Eagle's syndrome misdiagnosed as cranio-mandibular disorders. A retrospective study. *J Cranio-Maxillofac Surg.* 2020;48(10):1009–1017 [Fig. 7]. ISSN 1010-5182, https://doi.org/10.1016/j.jcms.2020.07.016, http://www.sciencedirect.com/science/article/pii/S1010518220301815)

long-lasting relief of the symptoms of Eagle syndrome as well as to avoid continued damage to the carotid artery (Fig. 12.10).

COMPLICATIONS AND PITFALLS

Eagle syndrome is an uncommon cause of facial pain. Because of the low incidence of Eagle syndrome relative to pain secondary to malignancy in this anatomic region, Eagle syndrome must be considered a diagnosis of exclusion. The clinician should always evaluate a patient with pain in this anatomic region for occult malignancy. Tumors of the larynx, hypopharynx, piriform sinus, and anterior triangle of the neck may manifest with clinical symptoms identical to those of Eagle syndrome (Fig. 12.11).

The major complications associated with this injection technique are related to trauma to the internal jugular and carotid artery. Hematoma formation and intravascular injection of local anesthetic with subsequent toxicity are common complications of this technique. Inadvertent blockade of the motor

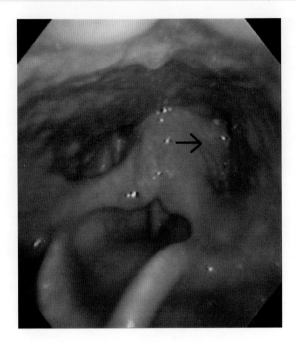

Fig. 12.11   Flexible laryngoscopy showed a left piriform sinus protruding tumor with an irregular surface *(arrow)*. (From Wang H-C, Leu Y-S, Tseng C-Y. Adenosquamous carcinoma of the hypopharynx. *J Cancer Res Pract*. 2018;5(2):81—83 [Fig. 2]. ISSN 2311-3006, https://doi.org/10.1016/j.jcrpr.2017.11.002.)

portion of the glossopharyngeal nerve can result in dysphagia secondary to weakness of the stylopharyngeus muscle. If the vagus nerve is inadvertently blocked, dysphonia secondary to paralysis of the ipsilateral vocal cord may occur. A reflex tachycardia secondary to vagal nerve block also is observed in some patients. Inadvertent block of the hypoglossal and spinal accessory nerves during glossopharyngeal nerve block results in weakness of the tongue and trapezius muscle.

HIGH-YIELD TAKEAWAYS

- The patient is afebrile, making an acute infectious etiology unlikely.
- The patient's symptomatology suggests pathology located in the anterolateral neck or hypopharynx.
- Eagle syndrome is a diagnosis of exclusion, given the disastrous consequences of missing a malignancy or foreign body of the hypopharynx.
- Plain radiographs and CT scanning of the neck is indicated in all patients thought to be suffering from Eagle syndrome.

Suggested Readings

Brassart N, Deforche M, Goutte A, et al. A rare vascular complication of Eagle syndrome highlight by CTA with neck flexion. *Radiol Case Rep.* 2020;15(8):1408–1412.

Finiels P-J, Batifol D. The treatment of occipital neuralgia: review of 111 cases. *Neurochirurgie.* 2016;62(5):233–240.

Janjua MB, Reddy S, El Ahmadieh TY, et al. Occipital neuralgia: a neurosurgical perspective. *J Clin Neurosci.* 2020;71:263–270.

Lee SYC, Lim MY, Loke SC, et al. Greater occipital nerve schwannoma—a rare cause of occipital neuralgia. *Otolaryngol Case Rep.* 2020;14:427–429.

Michiels TD, Marsman MJ, van Veen A, et al. Eagle syndrome: a unique cause of carotid bleeding. *JACC Case Rep.* 2020;2(3):449–453.

Waldman SD. Eagle syndrome. In: *Atlas of Uncommon Pain Syndromes.* 4th ed. Philadelphia: Elsevier; 2020:47–49.

Waldman SD. Eagle syndrome. In: *Pain Review.* 2nd ed. Philadelphia: Saunders; 2017: 216–217.

Waldman SD. Styloid process injection for Eagle syndrome. In: *Atlas of Pain Management Injection Techniques.* 4th ed. Philadelphia: Elsevier; 2017:32–35.

Waldman SD. Ultrasound guided injection technique for Eagle syndrome. In: *Comprehensive Atlas of Ultrasound-Guided Pain Management Injection Techniques.* 2nd ed. New York: Wolters Kluwer; 2020:95–103.

Brenda Brown

A 66-Year-Old Bookkeeper With Severe, Shocklike Facial Pain

- Learn the common causes of facial pain.
- Develop an understanding of the unique anatomy of the trigeminal nerve.
- Develop an understanding of the sensory innervation of the face.
- Develop an understanding of the causes of facial pain.
- Develop an understanding of the differential diagnosis of facial pain.
- Learn the clinical presentation of trigeminal neuralgia.
- Learn testing options to diagnose facial pain.
- Learn how to use physical examination to diagnose facial pain.
- Develop an understanding of the treatment options for the various types of facial pain.

Brenda Brown

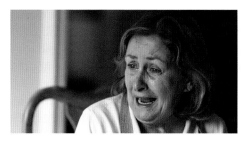

Brenda Brown is a 66-year-old book-keeper with the chief complaint of "horrible electric shocks in my face." Brenda stated that for the last 6 weeks, she has been experiencing electric shocks in her right jaw that "come out of nowhere and then go away as quick as they come." Brenda started crying and said, "Doctor, I just don't know how much more of this pain I can take! It's horrible, worse than anything you can imagine." Between sobs, she said," I wouldn't wish this pain on my worst enemy. I can't eat, drink, or clean my teeth. I'm living on lukewarm oatmeal and even that triggers the shocks." I asked Brenda if she had ever had anything like this before and she shook her head no. "Any fever or chills?" and again she shook her head no. "Is the pain there all of the time?" I asked. Brenda took a couple of deep breaths in an effort to calm down, then she said, "I am so sorry, Doctor, but I am just so played out. But to answer your question, the pain comes and goes. It hits me out of nowhere. Within a second or two, I am crying out in pain. My face jerks like it's trying to get away from the pain, and as quick as it comes, it is gone. Then if I sit quietly there is no pain; then out of nowhere, it hits again. It is relentless."

"Doctor, the pain can hit and wake me up from a sound sleep. If I roll over onto my right side, the touch of the pillow is all it takes to trigger the pain. I have been sleeping in my recliner for the last month. At first, I thought I had a bad tooth, but I went to the dentist and he said he thought the pain was in my nerves. I still have nightmares about the dentist examining me. It was like torture. But honestly, I would let him pull out all of my teeth without local if it would stop this pain." Brenda started crying again, and the crying triggered paroxysm of pain.

I worked to calm down Brenda, and then asked her to point with one finger to show me where it hurt the most. She pointed to the angle of the right mandi-ble, taking great care not to touch it. "Doctor, this is where the shocks hit, but I really can't tell where they come from. They come on so fast and with such force that I don't know which end is up. It takes all of my strength to keep from screaming."

I told Brenda that we would figure this out and that I would do everything in my power to stop the pain. I asked if I could examine her and she became upset again and said, "Doctor, please don't touch my jaw! Please don't. I can't take much more of this. Go ahead, but please don't touch my jaw!"

On physical examination, Brenda was afebrile. Her respirations were 18 and her pulse was 84 and regular. Her blood pressure was 148/94. Brenda's fundoscopic examination was normal as was the remainder of her eye examination. Taking care not to touch her, I had Brenda open her mouth, which triggered another paroxysm of pain. I didn't see any gross abnormalities, but her dental hygiene was pretty bad. Her cardiopulmonary examination was normal. I did not examine the thyroid or palpate for neck adenopathy in an effort to avoid triggering any more pain. Brenda's abdominal examination revealed no abnormal mass or organomegaly. There was no costovertebral angle (CVA) tenderness. There was no peripheral edema. Her low back examination was unremarkable. Visual inspection of the face was normal bilaterally. I noted that Brenda experienced facial tics with the paroxysms of pain. A careful neurologic examination of the upper and lower extremities revealed no evidence of peripheral or entrapment neuropathy. Her deep tendon reflexes were normal, and there were no pathologic reflexes or other abnormalities of the neurologic examination. I told Brenda that I was pretty sure I knew what was going on and that the good news was there were many treatment options to begin immediately. Brenda started crying again and kept saying, "Thank you, God. Thank you, God."

Key Clinical Points—What's Important and What's Not

THE HISTORY

- No history of previous facial pain
- No fever or chills
- Recent onset of unilateral facial pain characterized by electric shocklike pain centered at the angle of the right mandible
- Onset to peak of seconds to 1 minute
- Pain is episodic, with pain-free periods
- Pain triggered by swallowing, chewing, cleaning teeth
- Trigger areas in the third division of the trigeminal nerve on the right
- Recent normal dental examination
- Sleep disturbance
- High degree of anxiety regarding pain

THE PHYSICAL EXAMINATION

- Patient is afebrile
- Trigger areas in the third division of the trigeminal nerve on the right
- Facial tics associated with pain
- Poor dental hygiene
- Otherwise normal neurologic examination
- Normal fundoscopic examination
- No fever

OTHER FINDINGS OF NOTE

- Normal cardiovascular examination
- Normal pulmonary examination
- Normal abdominal examination
- No peripheral edema

 ## What Tests Would You Like to Order?

The following tests were ordered:
- Magnetic resonance imaging (MRI) of the brain with special attention to the brainstem
- Magnetic resonance angiography (MRA) of the cerebral circulation
- Erythrocyte sedimentation rate

TEST RESULTS

- MRI of the brain with special attention to the brainstem reveals a neurovascular conflict on the right side with the trigeminal nerve compressed between the supracerebellar artery and the petrosal vein (Fig. 13.1).
- MRA revealed a dolichoectatic basilar artery, touching the left trigeminal nerve (Fig. 13.2).
- Erythrocyte sedimentation rate was reported as 14 mm/hr.

 ## Clinical Correlation—Putting It All Together

What is the diagnosis?
Trigeminal neuralgia

The Science Behind the Diagnosis
ANATOMY

The trigeminal nerve is the fifth cranial nerve, and it derives its name from its three branches: the ophthalmic (V1), the maxillary (V2), and the mandibular (V3) (Fig. 13.3). The ophthalmic and maxillary nerves are comprised solely of sensory fibers, while the mandibular nerve has both sensory and motor fibers. The trigeminal nerve exits the pons as a single nerve root on each side of the pons. These bilateral nerve roots travel forward and laterally from the pons to form the gasserian ganglion (also known as the trigeminal ganglion), which is located in Meckel cave in the middle cranial fossa (Fig. 13.4). The canoe-shaped gasserian ganglion is bathed in cerebrospinal fluid and is surrounded by dura mater.

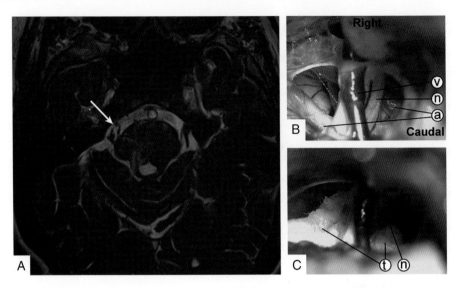

Fig. 13.1 Example of concordant (true positive) magnetic resonance imaging (MRI) and intraoperative findings. The patient is an elderly woman with right trigeminal neuralgia (TN) for the past 2 years unresponsive to medication. (A) MRI reveals a neurovascular conflict on the right side *(arrow)*. (B) Intraoperative photograph of the supracerebellar artery *(a)* ventral to the trigeminal nerve *(n)*, with the petrosal vein *(v)* lying posterior to the nerve. (C) Teflon sponge barrier (polytetrafluoroethene) *(t)* is inserted ventral to the nerve *(n)* from medial to lateral. The patient is relieved of TN. (From Hitchon PW, Bathla G, Moritani T, et al. Predictability of vascular conflict by MRI in trigeminal neuralgia. *Clin Neurol Neurosurg.* 2019;182:171–176 [Fig. 1]. ISSN 0303-8467, https://doi.org/10.1016/j.clineuro.2019.05.005, http://www.sciencedirect.com/science/article/pii/S0303846719301453)

The sensory fibers of the trigeminal nerve provide afferent light touch and proprioceptive and nociceptive functions, while the motor fibers of the mandibular nerve provide efferent innervation of the muscles of mastication, the myohyoid muscle, the anterior belly of the diagastric muscle, and the tensor typani and tensor veli palitini muscles. While the mandibular nerve is responsible for the light touch, proprioception, and pain and temperature sensation within its area of innervation, it does not transmit taste sensation, which is transmitted by the chorda tympani.

The ophthalmic division (V1) of the trigeminal nerve exits the cranial fossa via the superior orbital fissure and transmits sensory information from the scalp, forehead, upper eyelid, the conjunctiva and cornea of the eye, most of the nose except the nasal ala, the nasal mucosa, the frontal sinuses, and the dura and some intracranial vessels (Fig. 13.5). The maxillary division of the trigeminal nerve (V2) exits the cranial fossa via the foramen rotundum and transmits afferent sensory information from the lower eyelid and cheek, the nasal ala, the upper lip, upper dentition and gingiva, the nasal mucosa, the palate and roof of the pharynx, the maxillary, ethmoid and sphenoid sinuses, and

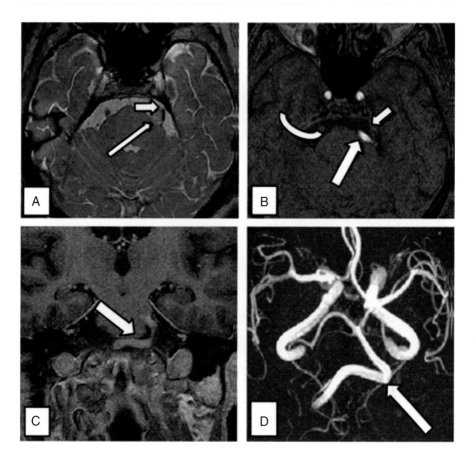

Fig. 13.2 A 54-year-old male with left trigeminal neuralgia. Magnetic resonance imaging (MRI) of the brain trigeminal protocol showing dolichoectatic basilar artery *(long arrows)*, touching the trigeminal nerve *(short arrows)*. (A) Axial constructive interference in steady state (CISS) of the cisteral portion. (B) MR angiography (MRA); note the relatively diminished caliber of the trigeminal nerve when compared to the contralateral side *(curved arrow)*. (C) Postcontrast series in coronal plane and (D) MRA clearly showing the dolichoectatic course of the basilar artery *(arrows)*. (From Geneidi EAS, Ali HI, Ghany WAA, et al. Trigeminal pain: potential role of MRI. *Egypt J Radiol Nucl Med*. 2016;47(4):1549–1555 [Fig. 6]. ISSN 0378-603X, https://doi.org/10.1016/j.ejrnm.2016.07.010, http://www.sciencedirect.com/science/article/pii/S0378603X16301140)

portions of the meninges. The mandibular division of the trigeminal nerve (V3) exits the cranial fossa via the foramen ovale and transmits sensory information from the lower lip, the lower dentition and gingiva, the chin and jaw (except the angle of the jaw, which is supplied by C2-C3), parts of the external ear, and parts of the meninges. The nerve also transmits sensory information from the dorsal aspect of the anterior two-thirds of the tongue and associated mucosa of the oral cavity.

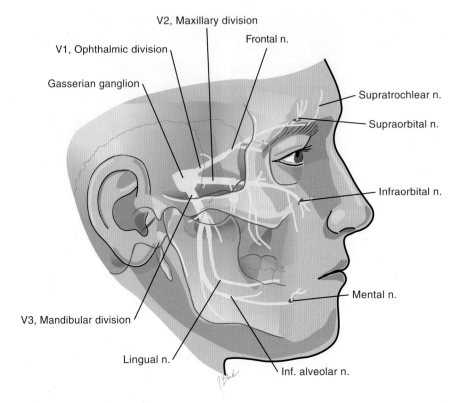

Fig. 13.3 The trigeminal nerve is the fifth cranial nerve, and it derives its name from its three branches: the ophthalmic (V1), the maxillary (V2), and the mandibular (V3). *n*, Nerve. (From Waldman S. *Atlas of Interventional Pain Management*. 5th ed. Philadelphia: Elsevier; 2021 [Fig. 9-2].)

CLINICAL SYNDROME

Trigeminal neuralgia occurs in many patients because of tortuous blood vessels that compress the trigeminal root as it exits the brainstem (see Fig. 13.1). Acoustic neuromas, cholesteatomas, aneurysms, angiomas, cysts, tumors, and bony abnormalities may also lead to compression of the nerve (Fig. 13.6). The severity of the pain produced by trigeminal neuralgia is rivaled only by that of cluster headache. Uncontrolled pain has been associated with suicide and should therefore be treated as an emergency. Attacks can be triggered by daily activities involving contact with the face, such as brushing the teeth, shaving, and washing (Fig. 13.7). Pain can be controlled with medication in most patients. Approximately 2% to 3% of patients with trigeminal neuralgia also have multiple sclerosis. Trigeminal neuralgia is also called tic douloureux.

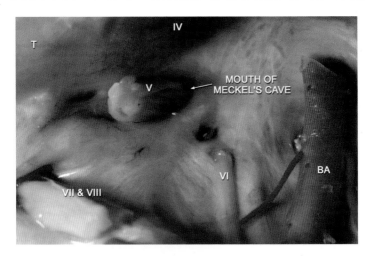

Fig. 13.4 Meckel cave and surrounding structures. Photograph of the mouth of Meckel cave, left side. *BA*, Basilar artery; *IV*, trochlear nerve; *T*, tentorium; *V*, trigeminal nerve; *VI*, abducens nerve; *VII*, facial nerve; *VIII*, vestibulocochlear nerve. (From Sabancı PA, Batay F, Civelek E, et al. Meckel's cave. *World Neurosurg.* 2011;76(3-4):335–341 [Fig. 3]. ISSN 1878-8750, https://doi.org/10.1016/j.wneu.2011.03.037, http://www.sciencedirect.com/science/article/pii/S187887501100369X)

SIGNS AND SYMPTOMS

Trigeminal neuralgia causes episodic pain afflicting the areas of the face supplied by the trigeminal nerve. The pain is unilateral in 97% of cases; when it does occur bilaterally, the same division of the nerve is involved on both sides. The second or third division of the nerve is affected in most patients, and the first division is affected less than 5% of the time. The pain develops on the right side of the face in 57% of unilateral cases. Trigeminal neuralgia occurs more commonly in women.

The pain of trigeminal neuralgia is characterized by paroxysms of electric shocklike pain lasting from several seconds to less than 2 minutes. The progression from onset to peak is essentially instantaneous. Patients with trigeminal neuralgia go to great lengths to avoid any contact with trigger areas. In contrast, persons with other types of facial pain, such as temporomandibular joint dysfunction, tend to rub the affected area constantly or apply heat or cold to it. Patients with uncontrolled trigeminal neuralgia frequently require hospitalization for rapid control of pain. Between attacks, patients are relatively pain free. A dull ache remaining after the intense pain subsides may indicate persistent compression of the nerve by a structural lesion. This disease is hardly ever seen in persons younger than 30 years unless it is associated with multiple sclerosis.

Patients with trigeminal neuralgia often have severe depression (sometimes to the point of being suicidal), with high levels of superimposed anxiety during

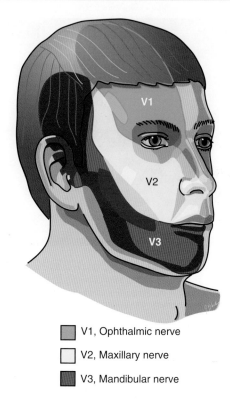

- ■ V1, Ophthalmic nerve
- □ V2, Maxillary nerve
- ■ V3, Mandibular nerve

Fig. 13.5   The sensory divisions of the trigeminal nerve. (From Waldman S. *Atlas of Interventional Pain Management.* 5th ed. Philadelphia: Elsevier; 2021 [Fig. 12-1]. 9780323654074.)

acute attacks. Both these problems may be exacerbated by the sleep deprivation that often accompanies painful episodes. Patients with coexisting multiple sclerosis may exhibit the euphoric dementia characteristic of that disease. Physicians should reassure persons with trigeminal neuralgia that the pain can almost always be controlled.

TESTING

All patients with a new diagnosis of trigeminal neuralgia should undergo MRI of the brain and brainstem, with and without gadolinium contrast medium, to rule out posterior fossa or brainstem lesions and demyelinating disease (see Fig. 13.1). MRA is also useful to confirm vascular compression of the trigeminal nerve by aberrant blood vessels (see Fig. 13.2). CT angiography may also be useful to clarify the role of aberrant blood vessels in the evolution of the patient's pain symptomatology (Fig. 13.8). Additional imaging of the sinuses should be considered if occult or coexisting sinus disease is a possibility. If the

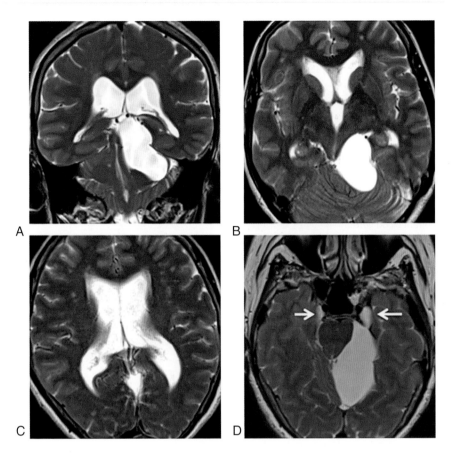

A   B

C   D

Fig. 13.6 Coronal T2-weighted magnetic resonance imaging revealed an arachnoid cyst at the cerebellopontine angle in contact with the trigone of the ipsilateral lateral ventricle in a 67-year-old patient with bilateral trigeminal neuralgia (A). The cyst extended into the quadrigeminal cistern of the left side (B), and associated obstructive hydrocephalus appeared on the axial section (C). Obvious dilation of both sides of Meckel cave *(arrows)* is observed on the axial section (D). (From Hayashi Y, Takata S, Iizuka H. Endoscopic treatment for arachnoid cyst at the cerebellopontine angle presenting with bilateral trigeminal neuralgia: case report and literature review. *Interdiscip Neurosurg.* 2020;22:100815 [Fig. 2]. ISSN 2214-7519, https://doi.org/10.1016/j.inat.2020.100815, http://www.sciencedirect.com/science/article/pii/S2214751920303765)

first division of the trigeminal nerve is affected, ophthalmologic evaluation to measure intraocular pressure and to rule out intraocular disease is indicated. Screening laboratory tests consisting of a complete blood count, erythrocyte sedimentation rate, and automated blood chemistry should be performed if the diagnosis of trigeminal neuralgia is in question. A complete blood count is required for baseline comparisons before starting treatment with carbamazepine (see "Treatment").

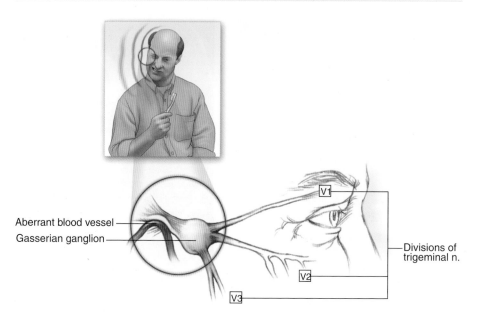

Aberrant blood vessel
Gasserian ganglion

Divisions of trigeminal n.

Fig. 13.7   Paroxysms of pain triggered by brushing the teeth in a patient with trigeminal neuralgia. *n*, Nerve. (From Waldman S. *Atlas of Common Pain Syndromes*. 4th ed. Philadelphia: Elsevier; 2019 [Fig. 10.2].)

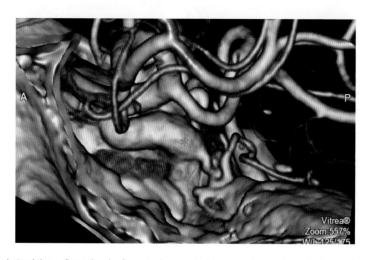

Fig. 13.8   Lateral three-dimensional reformatted computed tomography angiography image demonstrating origin of persistent trigeminal artery variant (PTAV) *(arrow)* from the cavernous segment of the inferior carotid artery (ICA) *(asterisk)*, proximal to the posterior genu. The tortuous PTAV is seen coursing posteriorly and eventually supplies the anterior ICA territory. (From Ling MM, Gupta M, Acharya J. Trigeminal neuralgia associated with a variant of persistent trigeminal artery. *Radiol Case Rep*. 2020;15(11):2225–2228 [Fig. 3]. ISSN 1930-0433, https://doi.org/10.1016/j.radcr.2020.08.057, http://www.sciencedirect.com/science/article/pii/S1930043320304568)

DIFFERENTIAL DIAGNOSIS

Trigeminal neuralgia is generally a straightforward clinical diagnosis that can be made on the basis of a targeted history and physical examination. Diseases of the eyes, ears, nose, throat, and teeth may all mimic trigeminal neuralgia or may coexist and confuse the diagnosis. Atypical facial pain is sometimes confused with trigeminal neuralgia, but it can be distinguished by the character of the pain: Atypical facial pain is dull and aching, whereas the pain of trigeminal neuralgia is sharp and neuritic (Table 13.1). Additionally, the pain of trigeminal neuralgia occurs in the distribution of the divisions of the trigeminal nerve, whereas the atypical facial pain does not follow any specific nerve distribution. Multiple sclerosis should be considered in all patients who present with trigeminal neuralgia before the fifth decade of life (Table 13.2).

TREATMENT

Drug therapy
Carbamazepine

Carbamazepine is considered first-line treatment for trigeminal neuralgia. In fact, a rapid response to this drug essentially confirms the clinical diagnosis. Despite the safety and efficacy of carbamazepine, some confusion and anxiety

TABLE 13.1 ■ **Comparison of Trigeminal Neuralgia, Glossopharyngeal Neuralgia, and Atypical Facial Pain**

	Trigeminal Neuralgia	Glossopharyngeal Neuralgia	Atypical Facial Pain
Location	Distribution of the trigeminal nerve—face	Distribution of the glossopharyngeal nerve—throat, tongue, tonsils, ear	Diffuse facial pain innonneuroanatomic distribution
Duration of Pain	Seconds to 1 min	Seconds to 1 min	Hours to constant
Character of Pain	Paroxysms of localized electric shocklike pain	Paroxysms of localized electric shocklike pain	Constant dull ache
Intensity of Pain	Severe	Severe	Mild to moderate
Provoking Factors	Talking, brushing teeth, touching trigger areas, shaving, drinking, eating	Swallowing, chewing, coughing, clearing throat, cold liquids	Stress, temperature changes, especially cold
Associated Symptoms	Facial tic or spasm	Bradycardia, syncope, arrythmia	Sensory abnormalities, including allodynia, temporomandibular joint dysfunction, bruxism
Prevalence	Rare	Extremely rare	Relatively common

TABLE 13.2 ■ Differential Diagnoses of Trigeminal Neuralgia

- Atypical facial pain
- Temporomandibular joint dysfunction
- Short-lasting unilateral neuralgiform headache
- Glossopharyngeal neuralgia
- Cluster headache
- Thunderclap headache
- Hemifacial spasm
- Multiple sclerosis
- Pain of dental origin
- Cerebral aneurysms
- Intracranial hemorrhage
- Acute herpes zoster
- Postherpetic neuralgia
- Primary stabbing headache
- Cavernous sinus syndromes
- Hydrocephalus
- Migraine headache
- Subarachnoid hemorrhage

surround its use. This medication, which may be the patient's best chance for pain control, is sometimes discontinued because of laboratory abnormalities erroneously attributed to it. Therefore baseline measurements consisting of a complete blood count, urinalysis, and automated blood chemistry profile should be obtained before starting the drug.

Carbamazepine should be initiated slowly if the pain is not out of control, with a starting dose of 100 to 200 mg at bedtime for 2 nights. The patient should be cautioned about side effects, including dizziness, sedation, confusion, and rash. The drug is increased in 100- to 200-mg increments given in equally divided doses over 2 days, as side effects allow, until pain relief is obtained or a total dose of 1200 mg/day is reached. Careful monitoring of laboratory parameters is mandatory to avoid the rare possibility of a life-threatening blood dyscrasia. At the first sign of blood count abnormality or rash, this drug should be discontinued. Failure to monitor patients who are taking carbamazepine can be disastrous because aplastic anemia can occur. When pain relief is obtained, the patient should be kept at that dosage of carbamazepine for at least 6 months before considering tapering the medication. The patient should be informed that under no circumstances should the drug dosage be changed or the drug refilled or discontinued without the physician's knowledge.

Gabapentin

In the uncommon event that carbamazepine does not adequately control a patient's pain, gabapentin may be considered. As with carbamazepine, baseline blood tests should be obtained before starting therapy, and the patient should be cautioned about potential side effects, including dizziness, sedation, confusion, and rash. The initial dose of gabapentin is 300 mg at bedtime for 2 nights. The drug is then increased in 300-mg increments given in equally divided doses over 2 days, as side effects allow, until pain relief is obtained or a total dose of 2400 mg/day is reached. At this point, if the patient has experienced only partial pain relief, blood values are measured, and the drug is carefully titrated upward using 100-mg tablets. Rarely is a dosage greater than 3600 mg/day required.

Baclofen

Baclofen may be of value in some patients who fail to obtain relief from carbamazepine or gabapentin. As with those drugs, baseline laboratory tests should be obtained before beginning baclofen therapy, and the patient should be warned about the same potential adverse effects. The patient starts with a 10-mg dose at bedtime for 2 nights; then the drug is increased in 10-mg increments given in equally divided doses over 7 days, as side effects allow, until pain relief is obtained or a total dose of 100 mg/day is reached. This drug has significant hepatic and central nervous system side effects, including weakness and sedation. As with carbamazepine, careful monitoring of laboratory values is indicated when using baclofen.

When treating individuals with any of these drugs, the physician should ensure that the patient knows that premature tapering or discontinuation of the medication may lead to the recurrence of pain, which will be more difficult to control.

Invasive therapy

Trigeminal nerve block

The use of trigeminal nerve block with local anesthetic and steroid is an excellent adjunct to drug treatment of trigeminal neuralgia. This technique rapidly relieves pain while medications are being titrated to effective levels. The initial block is carried out with preservative-free bupivacaine combined with methylprednisolone. Subsequent daily nerve blocks are performed in a similar manner, but using a lower dose of methylprednisolone. This approach may also be used to control breakthrough pain.

Retrogasserian injection of glycerol

The injection of small quantities of glycerol into the area of the gasserian ganglion can provide long-term relief for patients suffering from trigeminal neuralgia who have not responded to optimal drug therapy. This procedure should be performed only by a physician well versed in the problems and pitfalls associated with neurodestructive procedures (Fig. 13.9).

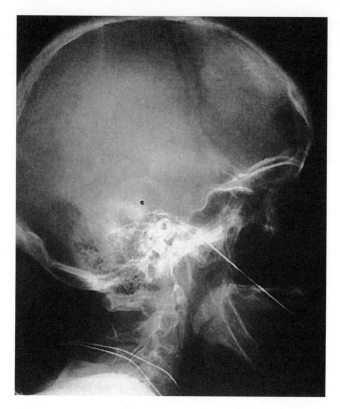

Fig. 13.9 Lateral fluoroscopic view of contrast injected into Meckel cave when performing gasserian ganglion block. (From Waldman SD. *Interventional Pain Management*. 2nd ed. Philadelphia: Saunders; 2001:320.)

Radiofrequency destruction of the gasserian ganglion

The gasserian ganglion can be destroyed by creating a radiofrequency lesion under biplanar fluoroscopic guidance. This procedure is reserved for patients in whom all the previously mentioned treatments for intractable trigeminal neuralgia have failed and who are not candidates for microvascular decompression of the trigeminal root.

Balloon compression of the gasserian ganglion

The insertion of a balloon by a needle placed through the foramen ovale into Meckel cave under radiographic guidance is a straightforward technique. Once the balloon is in proximity to the gasserian ganglion, it is inflated to compress the ganglion (Fig. 13.10). This technique has been shown to provide palliation of trigeminal neural pain in selected candidates in whom medication management has failed and who are not candidates for more invasive procedures.

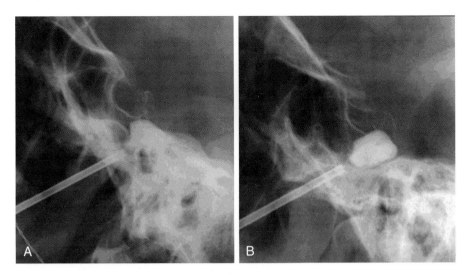

Fig. 13.10 Balloon compression of the gasserian ganglion. (A) Balloon placed within Meckel cave. (B) Lateral fluoroscopic view demonstrating inflated balloon within Meckel cave. (From Goerss SJ, Atkinson JL, Kallmes DF. Variable size percutaneous balloon compression of the gasserian ganglion for trigeminal neuralgia. *Surg Neurol.* 2009;71(3):388–390.)

Microvascular decompression of the trigeminal root

This technique, which is also called the Jannetta procedure, is the major neurosurgical treatment of choice for intractable trigeminal neuralgia. It is based on the theory that trigeminal neuralgia is in fact a compressive mononeuropathy. The operation consists of identifying the trigeminal root close to the brainstem and isolating the compressing blood vessel. A sponge is then interposed between the vessel and the nerve to relieve the compression and thus the pain (Fig. 13.11).

Gamma knife

Gamma knife is a painless outpatient procedure that uses the focused emission of gamma rays from a cobalt source to destroy the area anterior to the junction of the trigeminal nerve and the pons, the trigeminal nerve entry site immediately adjacent to the pons, the midposterior portion of the trigeminal nerve, or the cisternal segment of the trigeminal nerve. Complications include facial numbness and sensory deficit.

COMPLICATIONS AND PITFALLS

The pain of trigeminal neuralgia is severe and can lead to suicide. Therefore it must be considered a medical emergency, and strong consideration should be given to hospitalizing such patients. If a dull ache remains after the intense pain of trigeminal neuralgia subsides, this is highly suggestive of persistent

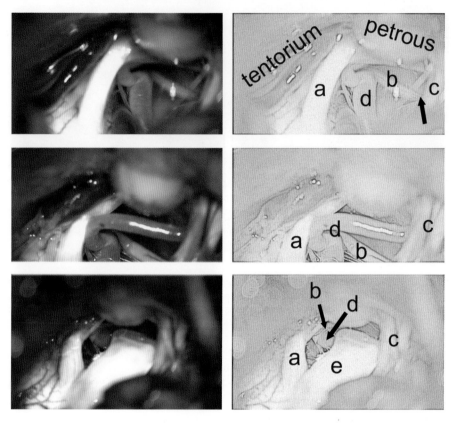

Fig. 13.11 Intraoperative microscope photographs during microvascular decompression of the right trigeminal nerve. *(Left column)* Three intraoperative microscope photographs at various stages of the procedure. *(Right column)* Identical faded photos to assist with labeling of structures. *(Top row)* The superior aspect of the right cerebellopontine angle has been exposed, revealing the tentorium, petrous, and trigeminal nerve *(a)* that is clearly compressed between a vein superiorly and a tortuous anterior inferior cerebellar artery (AICA) *(d)* inferiorly. The seventh and eighth nerve complex *(c)* can be seen inferiorly, toward the right of the frame. The sixth nerve *(b)* can be seen through the arachnoid after looping around the tortuous AICA as it descends inferiorly toward the Dorello canal *(arrow)*. *(Middle row)* The sixth nerve *(b)* is more clearly seen after arachnoid release, and severe compression of the trigeminal nerve *(a)* by the AICA *(d)* is more readily appreciated. *(Bottom row)* The AICA and its branches *(d)* have been mobilized inferiorly and stuck to the pons below the trigeminal nerve with Teflon and fibrin glue *(e)*. The loop of the abducent nerve around the AICA can be seen deep to the severely dented but now well-decompressed trigeminal nerve *(a)*. (From Borg A, Zrinzo L. Aberrant abducent nerve during microvascular decompression for trigeminal neuralgia. *World Neurosurg.* 2020;138:454–456 [Fig. 2]. ISSN 1878-8750, https://doi.org/10.1016/j.wneu.2020.03.115, http://www.sciencedirect.com/science/article/pii/S1878875020305866)

compression of the nerve by a structural lesion such as a brainstem tumor or schwannoma. Trigeminal neuralgia is hardly ever seen in persons younger than 30 years unless it is associated with multiple sclerosis, and all such patients should undergo MRI to identify demyelinating disease.

HIGH-YIELD TAKEAWAYS

- The patient is afebrile, making an acute infectious etiology unlikely.
- The patient's pain is unilateral and localized to the third division of the trigeminal nerve.
- The patient's pain is episodic with pain-free periods between the paroxysms of pain.
- The pain has an almost instantaneous onset to peak.
- The pain is electric shocklike in character.
- The patient has poor dental hygiene, suggesting the clinician should carefully assess the patient's nutritional and hydration status.
- The patient is quite stressed about the unremitting pain, and the risk of suicide remains ever present.
- Trigeminal neuralgia represents a true pain emergency.

Suggested Readings

Alper J, Shrivastava RK, Balchandani P. Is there a magnetic resonance imaging-discernible cause for trigeminal neuralgia? A structured review. *World Neurosurg.* 2017;98:89—97.

Bendtsen L, Zakrzewska JM, Heinskou TB, et al. Advances in diagnosis, classification, pathophysiology, and management of trigeminal neuralgia. *Lancet Neurol.* 2020;19 (9):784—796.

Donahue JH, Ornan DA, Mukherjee S. Imaging of vascular compression syndromes. *Radiol Clin North Am.* 2017;55(1):123—138.

Hitchon PW, Holland M, Noeller J, et al. Options in treating trigeminal neuralgia: experience with 195 patients. *Clin Neurol Neurosurg.* 2016;149:166—170.

Hoo JY, Sathasivam HP, Lau SH, et al. Symptomatic trigeminal neuralgia secondary to tumours: a case series. *J Oral Maxillofac Surg Med Pathol.* 2017;29(1):71—76.

Ling MM, Gupta M, Acharya J. Trigeminal neuralgia associated with a variant of persistent trigeminal artery. *Radiol Case Rep.* 2020;15(11):2225—2228.

Louges M-A, Kleiber J-C, Bazin A, et al. Efficacy of microsurgical vascular decompression in trigeminal neuralgia. *Eur Ann Otorhinolaryngol Head Neck Dis.* 2020;137(4):285—289.

Waldman SD. Gasserian ganglion block: balloon compression technique. In: *Atlas of Interventional Pain Management.* 5th ed. Philadelphia: Elsevier; 2021:44—48.

Waldman SD. Gasserian ganglion block. In: *Atlas of Interventional Pain Management.* 5th ed. Philadelphia: Elsevier; 2021:34—40.

Waldman SD. Gasserian ganglion block: radiofrequency lesioning. In: *Atlas of Interventional Pain Management.* 5th ed. Philadelphia: Elsevier; 2021:40—44.

Waldman SD. The trigeminal nerve. In: *Pain Review.* 2nd ed. Philadelphia: Elsevier; 2017: 376—377.

Waldman SD. Trigeminal neuralgia. In: *Atlas of Common Pain Syndromes.* 4th ed. Philadelphia: Elsevier; 2019:37—41.

Waldman SD. Trigeminal neuralgia. In: *Pain Review.* 2nd ed. Philadelphia: Elsevier; 2017: 207—209.

Tommy Flannagan

A 47-Year-Old Male With Severe Episodic Throat and Ear Pain

- Learn the common causes of facial pain.
- Develop an understanding of the unique anatomy of the glossopharyngeal nerve.
- Develop an understanding of the sensory innervation of the hypopharynx.
- Develop an understanding of the causes of ear pain.
- Develop an understanding of the differential diagnosis of throat and ear pain.
- Learn the clinical presentation of glossopharyngeal neuralgia.
- Learn testing options to diagnose glossopharyngeal neuralgia.
- Learn how to use physical examination to diagnose glossopharyngeal neuralgia.
- Develop an understanding of the treatment options for the various types of facial pain.

Tommy Flannagan

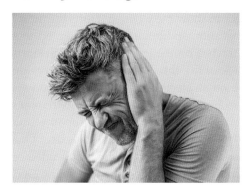

Tommy Flannagan is a 47-year-old male electrician with the chief complaint of, "I'm getting sharp pains in my throat and ear every time I swallow." Tommy stated that over the last 3 weeks, he had been having electric shocks that started in the back of his throat and then shot up into his ear. Tommy said that the pain would come out of nowhere and then go away as quick as it came. He said that it seemed like when he coughed or cleared his throat, it would trigger the pain, as did swallowing and sometimes chewing meat. "Tommy, is the pain on both sides or just on one side?" He replied, "It's always on the left, Doc. It's never on the right." Tommy went on to say that he had tried a heating pad and Tylenol, but the pain continued to get worse. I asked Tommy if had ever had anything like this before, and he shook his head no. I asked what made it better, and he said he had been "living off Campbell's tomato soup" to avoid triggering the pain, but that nothing really worked. I asked how he was sleeping, and he said he had taken to sleeping in his recliner because every time he rolled over onto his right side in bed, it triggered the pain that woke him. Tommy denied any fever or chills.

On physical examination, Tommy was afebrile. His respirations were 16 and his pulse was 68 and regular. His blood pressure was 118/72. His fundoscopic examination was normal. It took some convincing to get Tommy to open his mouth to let me examine his hypopharynx. I noted that Tommy still had his tonsils, but his dentition looked fine, and there was no obvious tumor or mass. When I touched the area just below the left tonsil with the tongue depressor, Tommy immediately cried out in pain and jerked away from me. I was glad that my fingers weren't in his mouth or he may have bitten them off. "Doc, warn me when you are going to do that again! It's really bad, and I need to have hold of something."

When I told him I wanted to take a look at his ears, he went nuts. "Doc, can you put me out before you look? I just don't know how much more of this pain I can take! It's horrible, worse than anything you can imagine. I did not know that anything could hurt this bad!" I said, "Let's start with the right ear and go from there. How about that?" Tommy was reluctant, but said, "Do what you have to do, Doc. I have to get better or I am done for. I am afraid this will hit when I am up on a ladder at work. What did I do to deserve this?" His right ear exam was normal, and with much convincing, I got a quick look at his left ear, which appeared completely normal. His cardiopulmonary examination and thyroid were normal. His abdominal examination revealed no abnormal mass or organomegaly. There was no costovertebral angle (CVA) tenderness. There was no peripheral edema. His low back examination was unremarkable.

I asked Tommy to point with one finger to show me where it "hurts the most" and with great care to avoid touching his submandibular area, he pointed to a point just below the mandible near the trachea on the left. "Doc, the pain starts way down deep in here—way at the back of my throat here—and it shoots up into my ear. Kinda ironic, isn't it? Here I am an electrician, and my own body is shocking me." A careful neurologic examination of the upper extremities revealed that there was no evidence of peripheral or entrapment neuropathy, and the deep tendon reflexes were normal. There were no pathologic reflexes. "One more question, Tommy. When you get the pain, do you ever get lightheaded or feel like you are going to pass out?" Tommy shook his head no and said, "Doc, never anything like that, but when it's really bad, I think about blowing my brains out. I guess it's a good thing that I don't have any guns." I told Tommy that I was pretty sure I knew what was going on and that we had a lot of treatment options to get on top of this pain. Tommy replied, "From your mouth to God's ears."

Key Clinical Points—What's Important and What's Not

THE HISTORY

- No history of previous facial pain
- No fever or chills
- Recent onset of unilateral throat and ear pain characterized by electric shocklike pain centered at the back of the throat on the left and radiating into the ipsilateral ear
- Onset to peak of seconds to 1 minute
- Pain is episodic with pain-free periods
- Pain triggered by swallowing, clearing of the throat, and chewing
- Trigger areas in the hypopharynx in the tonsillar area on the left
- Sleep disturbance
- High degree of anxiety regarding pain with suicidal ideation

THE PHYSICAL EXAMINATION

- Patient is afebrile
- Trigger areas in the hypopharynx on the left
- No obvious tumor or mass in the hypopharynx
- Normal ear examination bilaterally
- Normal neurologic examination
- Normal fundoscopic examination
- No fever

OTHER FINDINGS OF NOTE

- Normal cardiovascular examination, specifically no bradycardia or asystole
- Normal pulmonary examination
- Normal abdominal examination
- No peripheral edema
- Normal neurologic examination, motor and sensory examination
- No pathologic reflexes

 ## What Tests Would You Like to Order?

The following tests were ordered:
- Magnetic resonance imaging (MRI) of the brain with special attention to the brainstem
- Magnetic resonance angiography (MRA) of the cerebral circulation
- Electrocardiogram (ECG) with rhythm strip taken when patient triggers the pain
- Erythrocyte sedimentation rate

TEST RESULTS

- MRI of the brain with special attention to the brainstem revealed compression by the posterior inferior cerebellar artery as it crossed the glossopharyngeal nerve on the right (Fig. 14.1).

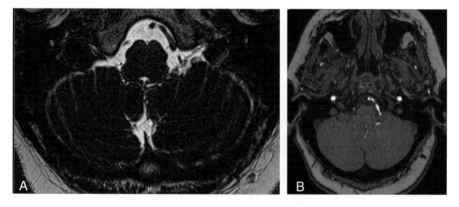

Fig. 14.1 (A) Magnetic resonance imaging (MRI) axial three-dimensional (3D) T2 SPACE. The arrow points to the posterior inferior cerebellar artery that crosses the glossopharyngeal nerve closely. (B) MRI axial 3D time of flight. The hyperintense line next to the brainstem is the thick posterior inferior cerebellar artery. *T2 SPACE*, Sampling perfection with application optimized contrasts using different flip angle evolution. (From den Hartog AW, Jansen E, Kal JE, et al. Recurrent syncope due to glossopharyngeal neuralgia. *Hear Case Rep.* 2017;3(1):73–77.)

- MRA confirmed the path of the inferior cerebellar artery as it crossed the glossopharyngeal nerve on the right.
- ECG with rhythm strip was within normal limits.
- The ESR is within normal limits.

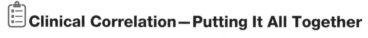 Clinical Correlation—Putting It All Together

What is the diagnosis?
Glossopharyngeal neuralgia

The Science Behind the Diagnosis
ANATOMY OF THE GLOSSOPHARYNGEAL NERVE

The glossopharyngeal nerve exits from the jugular foramen in proximity to the vagus and accessory nerves and the internal jugular vein and passes just inferior to the styloid process (Fig. 14.2). All three nerves lie in the groove between the internal jugular vein and internal carotid artery. The glossopharyngeal nerve

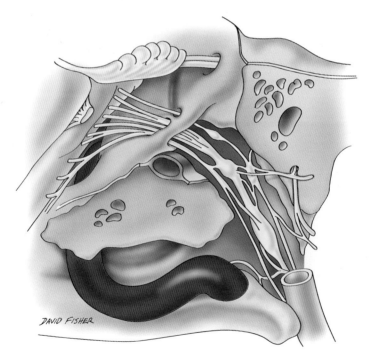

Fig. 14.2 Course of the glossopharyngeal nerve. Illustration of the glossopharyngeal nerve is schematized from the brainstem to the pharynx, with its various branches. (From Tubbs R, Rizk E, Shoja M, et al. *Nerves and Nerve Injuries*. London: Academic Press; 2015 [Fig. 5-1].)

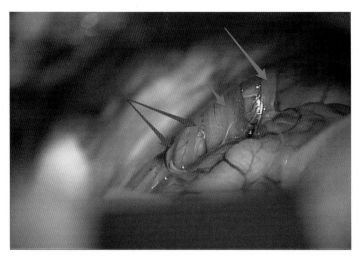

Fig. 14.3 Intracranial anatomy of glossopharyngeal nerve. Photograph of intraoperative intracranial view of the left glossopharyngeal nerve *(long blue arrow)* and the adjacent vagus nerve *(short blue arrow)*. Spinal and cranial accessory nerves *(red arrows)*. (From Tubbs R, Rizk E, Shoja M, et al. *Nerves and Nerve Injuries.* London: Academic Press; 2015 [Fig. 5.2].)

(cranial nerve IX) contains both motor and sensory fibers. The motor fibers innervate the stylopharyngeus muscle. The sensory portion of the nerve innervates the posterior third of the tongue, palatine tonsil, and the mucous membranes of the mouth and pharynx. Special visceral afferent sensory fibers transmit information from the taste buds of the posterior third of the tongue. The carotid sinus nerve, which is a branch of the glossopharyngeal nerve, carries information from the carotid sinus and body to help control blood pressure, pulse, and respiration. Parasympathetic fibers pass via the glossopharyngeal nerve to the otic ganglion. Postganglionic fibers from the ganglion carry secretory information to the parotid gland. The glossopharyngeal nerve lies in proximity to the vagus nerve as well as the spinal accessory nerve, which has significant clinical implications both in terms of cardiac arrythmias and compression by vascular structures (Figs. 14.3 and 14.4).

CLINICAL CONSIDERATIONS

Glossopharyngeal neuralgia is a rare condition characterized by paroxysms of pain in the sensory division of cranial nerve IX. Although the pain of glossopharyngeal neuralgia is similar to that of trigeminal neuralgia, it occurs 100 times less frequently. Glossopharyngeal neuralgia occurs more commonly in patients older than 50 years. The pain is located in the tonsil, laryngeal region, and posterior tongue (Fig. 14.5). The pain is unilateral in most patients, but it can occur bilaterally 2% of the time. Rarely, the pain of glossopharyngeal neuralgia is associated

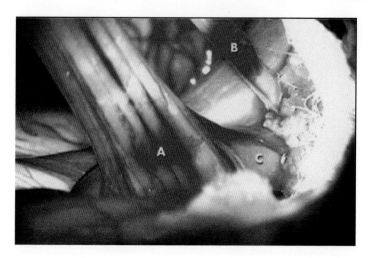

Fig. 14.4 Intraoperative photograph demonstrating compression of the glossopharyngeal and vagus nerves in a patient with glossopharyngeal neuralgia with associated syncope. *(A)* Vagus nerve (cranial nerve [CN] X). *(B)* Glossopharyngeal nerve (CN IX). *(C)* Large blood vessel (posterior inferior artery) causing compression. (From Horowitz M, Horowitz M, Ochs M, et al. Trigeminal neuralgia and glossopharyngeal neuralgia: two orofacial pain syndromes encountered by dentists. *J Am Dent Assoc.* 2004;135(10):1427–1433 [Fig. 2].)

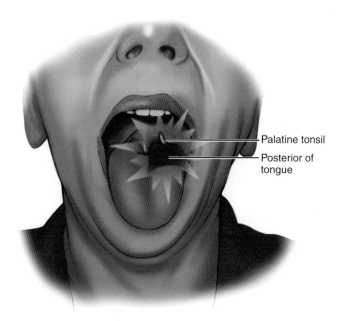

Palatine tonsil

Posterior of tongue

Fig. 14.5 The pain of glossopharyngeal neuralgia is in the distribution of cranial nerve IX. (From Waldman S. *Atlas of Uncommon Pain Syndromes.* 4th ed. Philadelphia: Elsevier; 2020 [Fig. 20-1].)

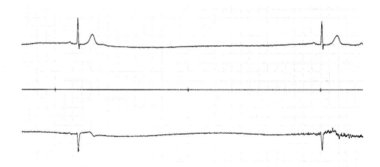

Fig. 14.6   Electrocardiogram of patient with glossopharyngeal neuralgia-induced syncope.

with bradyarrhythmias; in some patients, it is associated with syncope (Fig. 14.6). These cardiac symptoms are thought to be due to overflow of neural impulses from the glossopharyngeal nerve to the vagus nerve due to their proximity (see Fig. 14.3). Although rare, this unusual combination of pain and cardiac arrhythmia can be lethal. Facial tics and spasms can also be seen in combination with the pain of glossopharyngeal neuralgia (Fig. 14.7).

SIGNS AND SYMPTOMS

The pain of glossopharyngeal neuralgia is in the distribution of cranial nerve IX (Fig. 14.8; see Fig. 14.2). In some patients, overflow pain may occur in areas innervated by the trigeminal nerve, upper cervical segments, or both. The pain is neuritic and is unilateral in 98% of patients. It is often described as shooting or stabbing, with a severe intensity level. The pain of glossopharyngeal neuralgia is often triggered by swallowing, chewing, coughing, or talking. With the exception of trigger areas in the distribution of cranial nerve IX, the patient's neurologic examination should be normal. Because tumors at the cerebellopontine angle may produce symptoms identical to those of glossopharyngeal neuralgia, an abnormal neurologic examination is cause for serious concern (Fig. 14.9). Dull, aching pain that persists between the paroxysms of pain normally associated with glossopharyngeal neuralgia is highly suggestive of a space-occupying lesion and requires thorough evaluation.

TESTING

MRI of the brain and brainstem should be performed in all patients thought to have glossopharyngeal neuralgia. MRI of the brain provides the best information regarding the cranial vault and its contents. MRI is highly accurate and helps

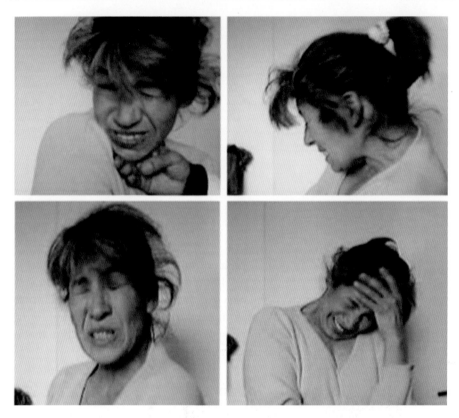

Fig. 14.7   Patient with hemifacial spasm associated with glossopharyngeal neuralgia. (From Abaroa L, Garretto NS. Meige's syndrome. *Reference Module in Neuroscience and Biobehavioral Psychology.* Elsevier; 2017 [Fig. 1]. ISBN 9780128093245, https://doi.org/10.1016/B978-0-12-809324-5.00666-0, http://www.sciencedirect.com/science/article/pii/B9780128093245006660)

identify abnormalities that may put the patient at risk for neurologic disasters secondary to intracranial and brainstem pathology, including tumors and demyelinating disease (Fig. 14.10; see Fig. 14.9). MRA may be helpful in identifying aneurysms responsible for neurologic symptoms. In patients who cannot undergo MRI, such as patients with pacemakers, computed tomography (CT) is a reasonable second choice.

Clinical laboratory tests consisting of complete blood cell count, automated chemistry profile, and erythrocyte sedimentation rate are indicated to rule out infection, temporal arteritis, and malignancy that may mimic glossopharyngeal neuralgia. Endoscopy of the hypopharynx with special attention to the piriform sinuses also is indicated to rule out occult malignancy. ECG with a rhythm strip taken during the trigger of pain is indicated in all patients thought to be suffering from glossopharyngeal neuralgia to rule out associated cardiac arrythmias, including asystole (see Fig. 14.6). Differential neural blockade of the glossopharyngeal

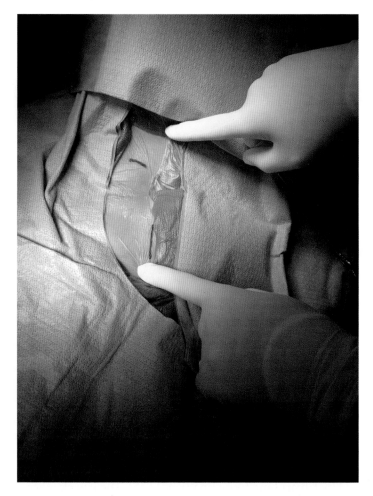

Fig. 14.8 Branches of the glossopharyngeal nerve. (From Tubbs R, Rizk E, Shoja M, et al. *Nerves and Nerve Injuries*. London: Academic Press; 2015 [Fig. 26.2].)

nerve may help strengthen the diagnosis of glossopharyngeal neuralgia (Fig. 14.11).

DIFFERENTIAL DIAGNOSIS

Glossopharyngeal neuralgia is generally a straightforward clinical diagnosis that can be made on the basis of a targeted history and physical examination. Diseases of the eye, ears, nose, throat, and teeth may mimic trigeminal neuralgia or may coexist and confuse the diagnosis (Table 14.1). Tumors of the hypopharynx, including the tonsillar fossa and piriform sinuses, may mimic the pain of

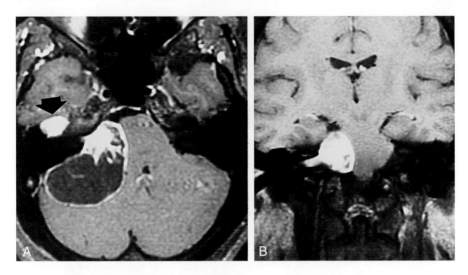

Fig. 14.9 Mixed cystic and solid acoustic nerve schwannoma in association with a solid schwannoma of the geniculate ganglion. (A) Axial enhanced image with fat saturation. A large mass with solid and cystic enhancing components is seen in the right cerebellopontine angle. A separate, solid erosive tumor is seen in the region of the right geniculate ganglion *(arrowhead)*. (B) Coronal enhanced image with fat saturation. The characteristic mushroom appearance of an intracanalicular acoustic schwannoma with extension into the adjacent cerebellopontine angle is well seen. This more anterior section through the internal auditory canal does not show the cystic portion of the tumor, but it does show the compression of the adjacent brainstem. (From Stark DD, Bradley WG Jr, eds. *Magnetic Resonance Imaging*. 3rd ed. St Louis: Mosby; 1999:1219.)

glossopharyngeal neuralgia, as may tumors at the cerebellopontine angle. Occasionally, demyelinating disease may produce a clinical syndrome identical to glossopharyngeal neuralgia, and so can compression of the glossopharyngeal nerve caused by Chiari I malformation (Fig. 14.12). The jaw claudication associated with temporal arteritis also sometimes confuses the clinical picture, as does trigeminal neuralgia.

TREATMENT

Pharmacologic treatment
Carbamazepine

Carbamazepine is considered first-line treatment for glossopharyngeal neuralgia. Rapid response to this drug essentially confirms a clinical diagnosis of glossopharyngeal neuralgia. Despite the safety and efficacy of carbamazepine compared with other treatments for glossopharyngeal neuralgia, much confusion and unfounded anxiety surround its use. This medication, which may be the patient's best chance for pain control, is sometimes discontinued because of laboratory abnormalities erroneously attributed to it. Baseline screening laboratory tests, consisting of a

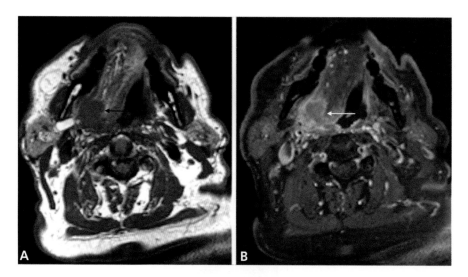

Fig. 14.10 Glossopharyngeal neuralgia caused by human papillomavirus—positive oropharyngeal squamous cell carcinoma. (A) Magnetic resonance imaging T1-weighted sequence demonstrates a hypointense mass at the right lateral aspect of tongue base *(black arrow)*. (B) The T1-weighted fat-suppressed sequence after gadolinium contrast reveals contrast enhancement of the mass suggestive of tumor *(white arrow)*. (From Sude A, Nixdorf DR, Grande AW. Human papillomavirus—positive oropharyngeal squamous cell carcinoma manifesting as glossopharyngeal neuralgia. *J Am Dent Assoc.* 2019;150(12):1059—1061 [Fig. A]. ISSN 0002-8177, https://doi.org/10.1016/j.adaj.2019.10.004, http://www.sciencedirect.com/science/article/pii/S0002817719307317)

complete blood cell count, urinalysis, and automated chemistry profile, should be obtained before starting the drug.

Carbamazepine should be started slowly, if the pain is not out of control, at a starting dose of 100 to 200 mg at bedtime for 2 nights; the patient should be cautioned regarding side effects, including dizziness, sedation, confusion, and rash. The drug is increased in 100- to 200-mg increments, given in equally divided doses over 2 days, as side effects allow, until pain relief is obtained or a total dose of 1200 mg per day is reached. Careful monitoring of laboratory parameters is mandatory to avoid the rare possibility of life-threatening blood dyscrasia. At the first sign of blood count abnormality or rash, this drug should be discontinued. Failure to monitor patients started on carbamazepine can be disastrous because aplastic anemia can occur. When pain relief is obtained, the patient should be kept at that dosage of carbamazepine for at least 6 months before considering tapering of this medication. The patient should be informed that under no circumstances should the dosage of drug be changed or the drug refilled or discontinued without the physician's knowledge.

Gabapentin

In the uncommon event that carbamazepine does not control a patient's pain adequately, gabapentin may be considered. As with carbamazepine, baseline

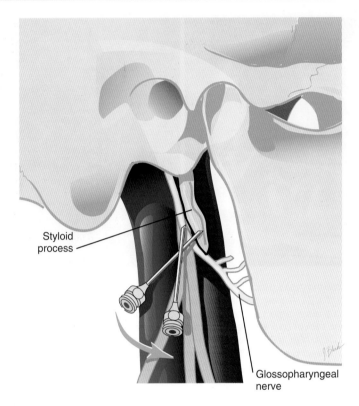

Fig. 14.11   Proper needle placement for glossopharyngeal nerve block. (From Waldman SD, ed. *Atlas of Interventional Pain Management Techniques*. 3rd ed. Philadelphia: Saunders; 2009.)

TABLE 14.1 ■ Differential Diagnosis of Glossopharyngeal Neuralgia

- Vascular compression
- Compression by tumor, cyst, or mass
- Eagle syndrome
- Trigeminal neuralgia
- Aneurysms of the carotid and vertebral arteries
- Arteriovenous malformations
- Tumors of the hypopharynx
- Infections of the hypopharynx
- Iatrogenic trauma to glossopharyngeal nerve following tonsillectomy, craniotomy, deep neck dissections
- Multiple sclerosis
- Temporal arteritis
- Stroke
- Chiari 1 malformation

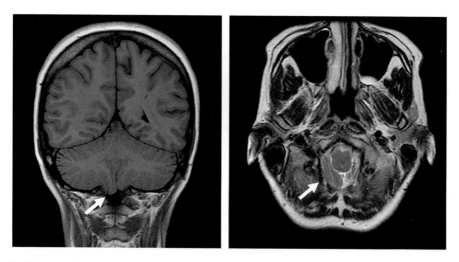

Fig. 14.12 Patient with glossopharyngeal neuralgia thought to be secondary to Chiari type I malformation. (A) Coronal fluid-attenuated inversion recovery magnetic resonance imaging (MRI), and (B) axial T2-weighted MRI showing an asymmetric tonsilar herniation on the right side compressing the posterolateral aspect of the medulla. The white arrows point to the descended tonsil. (From Ruiz-Juretschke F, García-Leal R, Garcia-Duque S, et al. Glossopharyngeal neuralgia in the context of a Chiari type I malformation. *J Clin Neurosci.* 2012;19(4):614—616 [Fig. 1]. ISSN 0967-5868, https://doi.org/10.1016/j.jocn.2011.05.040, http://www.sciencedirect.com/science/article/pii/S0967586811005327)

blood tests should be obtained before starting therapy. Gabapentin should be started with a 300-mg dose at bedtime for 2 nights; the patient should be cautioned about potential side effects, including dizziness, sedation, confusion, and rash. The drug is increased in 300-mg increments, given in equally divided doses over 2 days, as side effects allow, until pain relief is obtained or a total dose of 2400 mg per day is reached. At this point, if the patient has experienced partial pain relief, blood values are measured and the drug is carefully titrated using 100-mg tablets. More than 3600 mg per day is rarely required.

Baclofen
Baclofen has been reported to be of value in some patients who fail to obtain relief from carbamazepine and gabapentin. Baseline laboratory tests should be obtained before starting baclofen. The drug is started with a 10-mg dose at bedtime for 2 nights; the patient should be cautioned about potential adverse effects, which are the same as those of carbamazepine and gabapentin. The drug is increased in 10-mg increments, given in equally divided doses over 7 days, as side effects allow, until pain relief is obtained or a total dose of 80 mg daily is reached. This drug has significant hepatic and central nervous system side effects, including weakness and sedation. As with carbamazepine, careful monitoring of laboratory values is indicated during the initial use of this drug.

When treating patients with any of the drugs mentioned, the clinician should inform the patient that premature tapering or discontinuation of the medication may lead to the recurrence of pain. It becomes more difficult to control pain thereafter.

Interventional treatment

Glossopharyngeal nerve block

The use of glossopharyngeal nerve block with local anesthetic and a steroid serves as an excellent adjunct to drug treatment of glossopharyngeal neuralgia (see Fig. 14.11). This technique rapidly relieves pain while medications are being titrated to effective levels. The initial block is performed with preservative-free bupivacaine combined with methylprednisolone. Subsequent daily nerve blocks are done in a similar manner, substituting a lower dose of methylprednisolone. This approach also may be used to obtain control of breakthrough pain. Ultrasound guidance and the use of color Doppler to identify adjacent vasculature may improve the accuracy of needle placement and decrease the incidence of needle-induced trauma (Figs. 14.13, 14.14, and 14.15).

Radiofrequency destruction of the glossopharyngeal nerve

The destruction of the glossopharyngeal nerve can be carried out by creating a radiofrequency lesion under biplanar fluoroscopic guidance. This procedure is reserved for patients who have failed to respond to all the treatments mentioned for intractable glossopharyngeal neuralgia and who are not candidates for microvascular decompression of the glossopharyngeal root. Gamma knife ablation has also been used in this patient population.

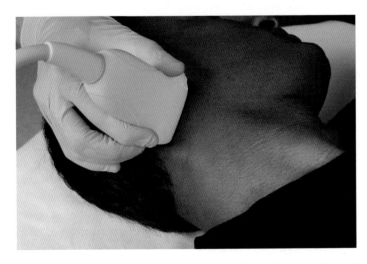

Fig. 14.13 Proper transverse placement of the linear ultrasound transducer over the previously identified styloid process.

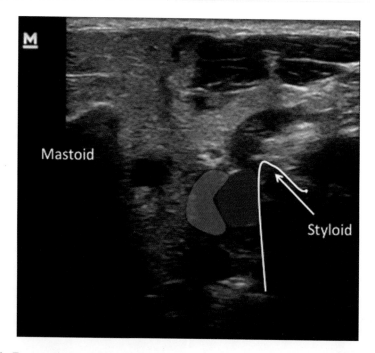

Fig. 14.14 Transverse ultrasound view of the styloid process, carotid artery, and jugular vein.

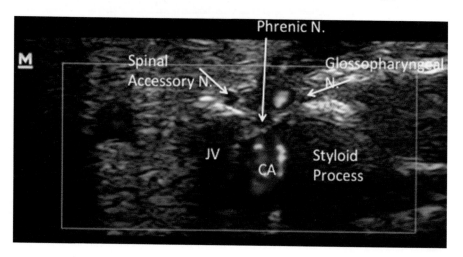

Fig. 14.15 Color Doppler image of the carotid artery and jugular vein. *CA*, Carotid artery; *JV*, jugular vein; *N*, nerve.

Microvascular decompression of the glossopharyngeal root

Microvascular decompression of the glossopharyngeal root, also referred to as the Jannetta procedure, is the major neurosurgical procedure of choice for intractable glossopharyngeal neuralgia. It is based on the theory that glossopharyngeal neuralgia is a compressive mononeuropathy analogous to trigeminal neuralgia. The operation consists of identifying the glossopharyngeal root close to the brainstem and isolating the offending compressing blood vessel. A sponge is interposed between the vessel and nerve, relieving the compression and the pain (Fig. 14.16).

Gamma knife. Gamma knife radiosurgery has been utilized in patients suffering from glossopharyngeal neuralgia who are too sick to undergo open neurosurgical microvascular decompression. Gamma knife is a painless outpatient procedure that uses the focused emission of gamma rays from a cobalt source to

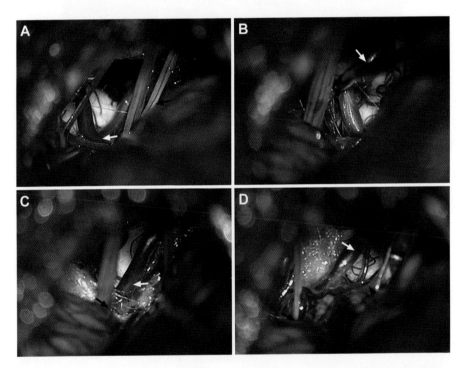

Fig. 14.16 Intraoperative photographs in a patient with coexistence of glossopharyngeal neuralgia and hemifacial spasm, revealing posterior inferior cerebellar artery (PICA) as offending vessel only. (A) Tortuous PICA *(white arrow)* was offending vessel, which compressed the root entry zone (REZ) of cranial nerve IX *(black arrow)*. (B) The PICA *(white arrow)* was removed from the REZ of the cranial nerve IX *(black arrow)*. (C) Teflon pads were inserted between the REZ of cranial nerve IX *(black arrow)* and the PICA *(white arrow)*. (D) The PICA *(white arrow)* was also compressed onto the REZ of cranial nerve VII *(black arrowhead)*. The PICA *(white arrow)* had been removed from the REZ of both cranial nerve IX *(black arrow)* and cranial nerve VII *(black arrowhead)*. (From Liu J, Shen Y, Jiang B, et al. Ameliorating effect of microvascular decompression on patients with coexistence of hemifacial spasm and glossopharyngeal neuralgia: a retrospective study. *World Neurosurg.* 2020;133:e62—e67 [Fig. 3]. ISSN 1878-8750, https://doi.org/10.1016/j.wneu.2019.08.069, http://www.sciencedirect.com/science/article/pii/S1878875019322247)

destroy an area in proximity to the glossopharyngeal nerve. Complications include sensory deficit and weakness of the stylopharyngeus muscle of the pharynx.

COMPLICATIONS AND PITFALLS

The pain of glossopharyngeal neuralgia is severe and can lead to suicide; therefore it must be considered a medical emergency, and strong consideration should be given to hospitalizing such patients. If a dull ache remains after the intense, paroxysmal pain of glossopharyngeal neuralgia subsides, this is highly suggestive of persistent compression of the nerve by a structural lesion such as a brainstem tumor or schwannoma. Glossopharyngeal neuralgia is almost never seen in persons younger than 30 years unless it is associated with multiple sclerosis, and all such patients should undergo MRI to identify demyelinating disease.

The major complications associated with glossopharyngeal nerve block are related to trauma to the internal jugular and carotid artery. Hematoma formation and intravascular injection of local anesthetic with subsequent toxicity are significant problems for the patient. Blockade of the motor portion of the glossopharyngeal nerve can result in dysphagia secondary to weakness of the stylopharyngeus muscle. If the vagus nerve is inadvertently blocked, as it often is during glossopharyngeal nerve block, dysphonia secondary to paralysis of the ipsilateral vocal cord may occur. Reflex tachycardia secondary to vagal nerve block is also observed in some patients. Inadvertent block of the hypoglossal and spinal accessory nerves during glossopharyngeal nerve block will result in weakness of the tongue and trapezius muscle.

The glossopharyngeal nerve is susceptible to trauma from the needle, hematoma, or compression during injection procedures. Such complications, although usually transitory, can be quite upsetting to the patient. Although uncommon, risk for infection is ever present, especially in patients who have cancer and are immunocompromised. Early detection of infection is crucial to avoiding potentially life-threatening sequelae.

HIGH-YIELD TAKEAWAYS

- The patient is afebrile, making an acute infectious etiology unlikely.
- The patient's pain is unilateral and localized to the distribution of the glossopharyngeal nerve.
- The patient's pain is episodic, with pain-free periods between the paroxysms of pain.
- The pain has an almost instantaneous onset to peak.

(Continued)

- The pain is electric shocklike in character.
- The clinician should carefully assess the nutritional and hydration status of all patients suffering from glossopharyngeal neuralgia.
- The patient is quite stressed about the unremitting pain, and the risk of suicide remains ever present.
- The clinician should take the suicide ideations seriously in this clinical setting.
- Glossopharyngeal neuralgia represents a true pain emergency.

Suggested Readings

Albahkaly S, Alshehabi M, Al-Shmasi HS, et al. Reappraisal of glossopharyngeal neuralgia. *Interdiscip Neurosurg.* 2018;11:34—36.

den Hartog AW, Jansen W, Kal JE, et al. Recurrent syncope due to glossopharyngeal neuralgia. *Hear Case Rep.* 2017;3(1):73—77.

Liu J, Shen Y, Jiang B, et al. Ameliorating effect of microvascular decompression on patients with coexistence of hemifacial spasm and glossopharyngeal neuralgia: a retrospective study. *World Neurosurg.* 2020;133:e62—e67.

Sude A, Nixdorf DR, Grande AW. Human papillomavirus—positive oropharyngeal squamous cell carcinoma manifesting as glossopharyngeal neuralgia. *J Am Dent Assoc.* 2019;150(12):1059—1061.

Waldman SD, ed. *Atlas of Interventional Pain Management.* 5th ed. Philadelphia: Elsevier; 2021:103—107.

Waldman SD. Glossopharyngeal neuralgia. In: *Atlas of Uncommon Pain Syndromes.* 4th ed. Philadelphia: Elsevier; 2020:62—66.

Waldman SD. Ultrasound guided glossopharyngeal nerve block. In: *Comprehensive Atlas of Ultrasound Guided Pain Management Injection Techniques.* 2nd ed. New York: Wolters Kluwer; 2020:105—111.

Heather Shepard

A 52-Year-Old Editor With Aching Jaw Pain and a Clicking Sensation

- Learn the common causes of facial pain.
- Develop an understanding of the unique anatomy of the temporomandibular joint.
- Develop an understanding of the sensory innervation of the face.
- Develop an understanding of the causes of facial pain.
- Develop an understanding of the differential diagnosis of facial pain.
- Learn the clinical presentation of temporomandibular joint pain.
- Learn testing options to diagnose facial pain.
- Learn how to use physical examination to diagnose facial pain.
- Develop an understanding of the treatment options for the various types of facial pain.

Heather Shepard

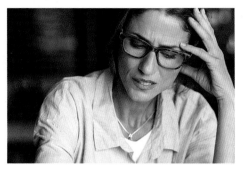

Heather Shepard is a 52-year-old editor with the chief complaint of "jaw pain that radiates into the ear." Heather was a longstanding patient and was one of the most uptight people that I had ever met. If you looked up "tense" in Wikipedia, you would see a picture of Heather. Over the years I had seen Heather for tension-type headaches, peptic ulcer, dysfunctional bowel, and insomnia. Stress had certainly taken its toll on Heather's health. Today, Heather was complaining of pain in her jaw. "Doctor, it feels like there is something wrong with my jaw. It is always clicking, and it hurts when I open and close my mouth." Heather went on to say that the pain was really driving her crazy. "It seems like I wake up with an achy jaw and by the end of the day, I just want to scream. It feels like someone hit me in the jaw with a baseball bat, like there should be a great big bruise there, but I look and there is nothing to see. I went to the dentist to see if there was something wrong with my teeth. The dentist took one look and said that I was grinding my teeth. The dentist then asked me if I was upset about anything. If I kept grinding my teeth, I would end up with dentures. That really made me mad. Like this is all in my head. So, I told her 'thanks, but no thanks,' and got the hell out of there. You don't have the name of a good dentist, do you?"

I asked Heather how long she had the jaw pain and she said, "You know, I've had the headaches you treated me for about as long as I can remember, but this jaw pain has come on gradually over the last 5 or 6 months. I can't really figure out what brought the pain on, but it is really driving me crazy." She said that other than the tightness around her head and her neck ache, she did not have any other symptoms that went along with her jaw pain.

I asked Heather if she had identified anything that triggered her jaw pain and she immediately shook her head no. I asked Heather if she had any other symptoms that went along with her jaw pain and she said that when she yawned or opened her mouth very wide, she would feel a clicking sensation. I asked if she was having any associated neck pain, and Heather said, "By the end of the day, I just want someone to give me a neck massage. I feel like the neck and headaches and jaw pain all go together. I feel like I am always clenching my teeth. I don't know why. I guess it's just become a habit."

I asked her what made it better, and she said, "I've tried all of the usual over-the-counter medications like Excedrin Migraine and Advil, but they really upset my stomach, so I can't take them very often. Remember those ulcers? Sometimes a heating pad and a glass of wine seem to help a little."

I asked Heather to use one finger to point at the spot where it hurt the most, and she pointed to her temporomandibular joint (TMJ) on the left. I asked her what the pain was like: an ache, sharp, stabbing, burning? She immediately said, "It's a deep, achy kind of feeling. Once in a while when my jaw clicks, I can feel it up in my ear, but not every time." I asked whether the jaw pain was on both sides or just one side, and she said it was always on the left, never on the right. I asked Heather from the time that she knew she was going to get the jaw pain until the time it was at its worst, was it a period of seconds, minutes, or hours. She responded, "It is always at least a few hours to a day before it is at its worst. But most days it is there when I wake up. It seems to get worse as the day goes on. As you know, my sleep has never been great, but this jaw pain sure hasn't helped."

On physical examination, Heather was afebrile. Her respirations were 16 and her pulse was 78 and regular. Her blood pressure was 126/80. There were no cranial abnormalities, and her eye, nose, and throat examination were completely normal, as was her fundoscopic examination. I could feel no mandibular mass, but a click was present on palpation of the TMJ when I had Heather open and close her mouth. I was shocked at the condition of Heather's teeth. Heather had broken off the occlusal surfaces of the teeth, presumably from bruxism (Fig. 15.1). Heather's cervical paraspinous muscles were tender to deep palpation, but no myofascial trigger points were identified. Her cardiopulmonary examination was normal, as was her thyroid. Her abdominal examination revealed no abnormal mass or organomegaly, and no rebound tenderness was

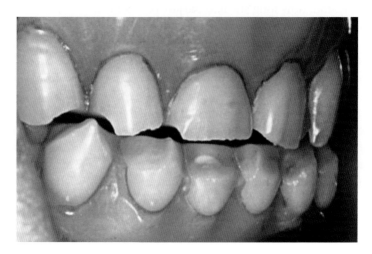

Fig. 15.1 Damage to the occlusal surfaces secondary to bruxism. (From Johansson A, Omar R, Carlsson GE. Bruxism and prosthetic treatment: a critical review. *J Prosthodont Res.* 2011;55(3):127–136 [Fig. 10]. ISSN 1883-1958, https://doi.org/10.1016/j.jpor.2011.02.004, http://www.sciencedirect.com/science/article/pii/S1883195811000387)

present. There was no costovertebral angle (CVA) tenderness. There was no peripheral edema. A careful neurologic examination of the upper and lower extremities revealed no evidence of weakness, lack of coordination, peripheral or entrapment neuropathy, and her deep tendon reflexes were normal. No pathologic reflexes were identified. Heather's mental status exam was within normal limits, but I was again struck by the high level of anxiety Heather displayed.

Key Clinical Points—What's Important and What's Not

THE HISTORY

- History of episodic tension-type headache
- Unilateral jaw pain
- Opening and closing of the mouth causes a clicking sensation with pain that radiates into the ipsilateral ear
- Jaw pain associated with nuchal pain and headache
- Character of the pain of headache was aching in nature, without throbbing
- Significant sleep disturbance
- Patient denies fever or chills
- Patient admits to clenching the jaw
- Headache associated with work stress

THE PHYSICAL EXAMINATION

- Patient is afebrile
- Clicking of the TMJ with opening and closing of mouth
- Broken teeth thought to be secondary to bruxism (see Fig. 15.1)
- Normal fundoscopic exam
- Examination of the cranium is normal
- Neurologic exam is normal
- Tenderness of the paraspinous muscles without myofascial trigger points

OTHER FINDINGS OF NOTE

- Normal cardiovascular examination
- Normal pulmonary examination
- Normal abdominal examination
- No peripheral edema
- Normal upper and lower extremity neurologic examination, motor and sensory examination

What Tests Would You Like to Order?

The following tests were ordered:
- Radiographs of the TMJs
- Arthrography of the TMJs
- Magnetic resonance imaging (MRI) of the TMJs

TEST RESULTS

- Radiographs of the TMJs revealed irregularity of surface (erosion) on upper portion of left condyle, indicating osteoarthritis (Fig. 15.2).
- Arthrography of the TMJs revealed intraarticular disc dislocation (Fig. 15.3).
- MRI of the TMJs revealed osteoarthritis and disc displacement (Fig. 15.4).

 Clinical Correlation—Putting It All Together

What is the diagnosis?
Temporomandibular joint pain

The Science Behind the Diagnosis
ANATOMY

The temporomandibular joint is a true joint divided into an upper and a lower synovial cavity by a fibrous articular disk. In health, the disc and muscles allow

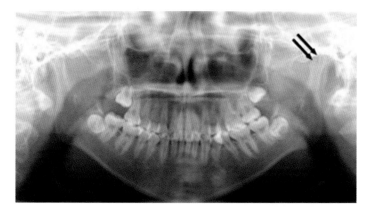

Fig. 15.2 Panoramic radiograph. Irregularity of surface (erosion) *(black arrows)* is seen on upper portion of left condyle, indicating osteoarthritis. However, patient did not complain of pain in left temporomandibular joint. (From Sano T, Yajima A, Otonari-Yamamoto M, et al. Interpretation of images and discrepancy between osteoarthritic findings and symptomatology in temporomandibular joint. *Jap Dent Sci Rev.* 2008;44(1):83–89 [Fig. 2].)

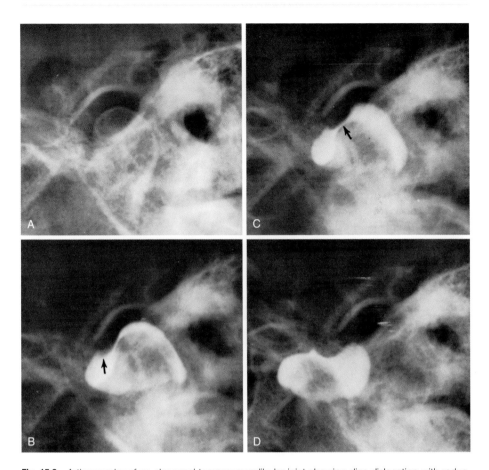

Fig. 15.3 Arthrography of an abnormal temporomandibular joint showing disc dislocation with reduction in a 20-year-old woman with clicking and intermittent pain. (A) Magnification transcranial radiograph with the mouth closed shows normal osseous anatomy and isocentric condyle position in the mandibular fossa. (B) With the mouth closed, contrast agent fills the inferior joint space and outlines the undersurface of the disc. The posterior band of the disc is located anterior to the condyle *(arrow)* and bulges prominently in the anterior recess. This appearance is diagnostic of anterior dislocation of the disc. (C) With the mouth half open, contrast agent has been redistributed, and the condyle has moved onto the posterior band *(arrow)*, which is now compressed between the condyle and the eminence. (D) With the mouth fully open, the condyle has translated anterior to the eminence; in so doing, it has crossed the prominent, thick posterior band and is causing a click. The posterior band is now in a normal position posterior to the condyle. (From Resnick D. *Diagnosis of Bone and Joint Disorders*. 4th ed. Philadelphia: Saunders; 2002:1723.)

the joint, muscles, and articular disc to move in concert (Figs. 15.5 and 15.6). The internal derangement of this disc may result in pain and TMJ dysfunction, but extracapsular causes of TMJ pain are much more common. The joint space between the mandibular condyle and the glenoid fossa of the zygoma may be injected with small amounts of local anesthetic and corticosteroid. The TMJ is innervated by branches of

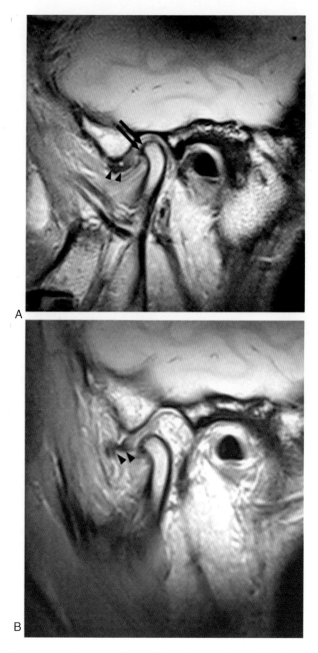

Fig. 15.4 Magnetic resonance images. Parasagittal proton density-weighted closed-mouth image (A) shows anterior osteophyte of condyle *(black arrows)*. Disc *(black arrowheads)* is anterior of condyle. On mouth opening (B), disc *(black arrows)* remained anterior. This was consistent with osteoarthritis associated with disk displacement without reduction. (From Sano T, Yajima A, Otonari-Yamamoto M, et al. Interpretation of images and discrepancy between osteoarthritic findings and symptomatology in temporomandibular joint. *Jap Dent Sci Rev.* 2008;44(1):83–89 [Fig. 3]. ISSN 1882-7616, https://doi.org/10.1016/j.jdsr.2008.02.001, http://www.sciencedirect.com/science/article/pii/S1882761608000112)

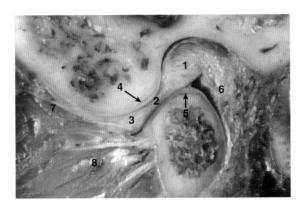

Fig. 15.5 Anatomic section through a temporomandibular joint. *1*, Pars posterior; *2*, pars intermediate; *3*, pars anterior; *4 and 5*, fibrocartilage covering the condyle and fossa; *6*, inferior lamina of the posterior attachment; *7 and 8*, superior and inferior head of the lateral pterygoid muscle. (Courtesy of Dr. Hans Ulrich Luder.)

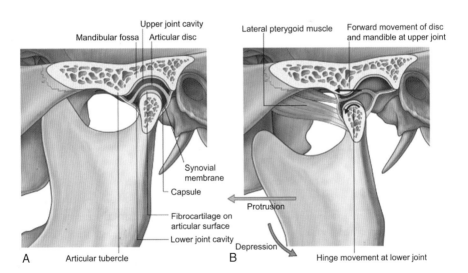

Fig. 15.6 Opening and closing of the temporomandibular joint. (A) Temporomandibular joint in closed position. (B) Temporomandibular joint in open position. (From Yin CS, Lee YJ, Lee YJ. Neurological influences of the temporomandibular joint. *J Bodywork Move Ther.* 2007;11(4):285–294 [Fig. 1]. ISSN 1360-18592, https://doi.org/10.1016/j.jbmt.2006.11.007, http://www.sciencedirect.com/science/article/pii/S1360859206001173)

the mandibular nerve. The muscles involved in jaw movement that have the potential to contribute to TMJ dysfunction often include the temporalis, masseter, and external and internal pterygoid and may include the trapezius and sternocleidomastoid (Fig. 15.7). Trigger points may be identified when these muscles are palpated.

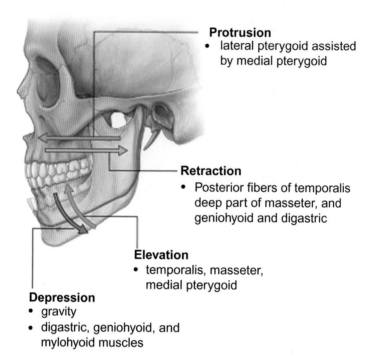

Protrusion
- lateral pterygoid assisted by medial pterygoid

Retraction
- Posterior fibers of temporalis deep part of masseter, and geniohyoid and digastric

Elevation
- temporalis, masseter, medial pterygoid

Depression
- gravity
- digastric, geniohyoid, and mylohyoid muscles

Fig. 15.7 Movement of the jaw. (From Yin CSK, Lee YJK, Lee YJ. Neurological influences of the tempo-romandibular joint. *J Bodyw Mov Ther.* 2007;11(4):285–294.)

CLINICAL SYNDROME

TMJ dysfunction (also known as myofascial pain dysfunction of the muscles of mastication) is characterized by pain in the joint itself that radiates into the mandible, ear, neck, and tonsillar pillars. The pain of TMJ dysfunction is made worse by chewing, speaking, or opening the mouth wide. Clicking, grating, and popping sensations often accompany the pain as does a tired feeling in the ipsilateral face.

Internal derangement of this disc may result in pain and TMJ dysfunction, but extracapsular causes of TMJ pain are much more common (Table 15.1). Rarely, the TMJ may lock, making it difficult to open or close the mouth.

SIGNS AND SYMPTOMS

Headache often accompanies the pain of TMJ dysfunction and is clinically indistinguishable from tension-type headache. Stress is often the precipitating factor or an exacerbating factor in the development of TMJ dysfunction (Fig. 15.8). A

TABLE 15.1 ▪ Causes and Mimics of Temporomandibular Joint Pain

- Intraarticular disorders
  - Osteoarthritis
  - Rheumatoid arthritis
  - Psoriatic arthritis
  - Ankylosing spondylitis
  - Reiter syndrome
  - Crystal arthropathies
- Intraarticular disc derangement
  - Disc displacement
  - Disc tearing
- Trauma
  - Intraarticular hemorrhage
  - Contusion
  - Bruising
- Temporal arteritis
- Tumor
- Infection
- Congenital disorders
- Postradiation fibrosis
- Trismus
- Reflex sympathetic dystrophy of the face
- Disorders involving muscles of mastication
  - Fibromyalgia
  - Myositis
  - Tenosynovitis
  - Muscle spasm
  - Bruxism

history of bruxism or jaw clenching is often present. Dental malocclusion may also play a role in its evolution. Internal derangement and arthritis of the TMJ may manifest as clicking or grating when the mouth is opened and closed. If the condition is untreated, the patient may experience increasing pain in the aforementioned areas as well as limitation of jaw movement and mouth opening.

Trigger points may be identified when palpating the muscles involved in TMJ dysfunction. Crepitus on range of motion of the joint suggests arthritis rather than dysfunction of myofascial origin. In severe cases, deviation of the mandible may occur (Fig. 15.9).

TESTING

Radiographs of the TMJ are usually within normal limits in patients suffering from TMJ dysfunction, but they may be useful to help identify inflammatory or degenerative arthritis of the joint as well as crystal deposition diseases (see Fig. 15.2). Arthroscopy and arthroscopy of the joint can help the clinician identify derangement of the disc as well as other abnormalities of the joint itself (Fig. 15.10).

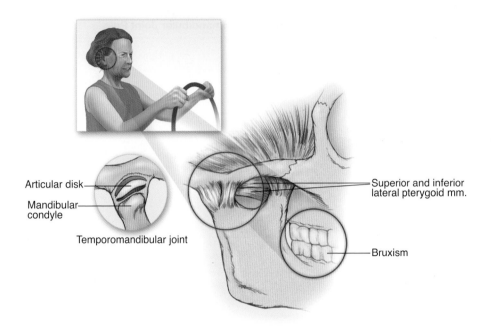

Fig. 15.8 Stress is often a trigger for temporomandibular joint dysfunction. *mm.:* muscles. (From Waldman S. *Atlas of Common Pain Syndromes*. 4th ed. Philadelphia: Elsevier; 2019 [Fig. 11-1].)

Computerized tomography, ultrasound imaging, and MRI may provide more detailed information regarding the condition of the disc and articular surface and should be considered in complicated cases (Fig. 15.11; see Fig. 15.4). A complete blood count, erythrocyte sedimentation rate, and antinuclear antibody testing are indicated if inflammatory arthritis or temporal arteritis is suspected. Injection of the joint with small amounts of local anesthetic can serve as a diagnostic maneuver to determine whether the TMJ is in fact the source of the patient's pain (Fig. 15.12). In select cases, arthrotomy and exploration of the joint may be indicated as both a diagnostic and therapeutic maneuver (Fig. 15.13).

DIFFERENTIAL DIAGNOSIS

The clinical symptoms of TMJ dysfunction may be confused with pain of dental or sinus origin or may be characterized as atypical facial pain (see Table 15.1). With careful questioning and physical examination, however, the clinician can usually distinguish these overlapping pain syndromes. Tumors of the zygoma and mandible, as well as retropharyngeal tumors, may produce ill-defined pain attributed to the TMJ, and these potentially life-threatening diseases must be excluded in any patient with facial pain. Reflex sympathetic dystrophy of the

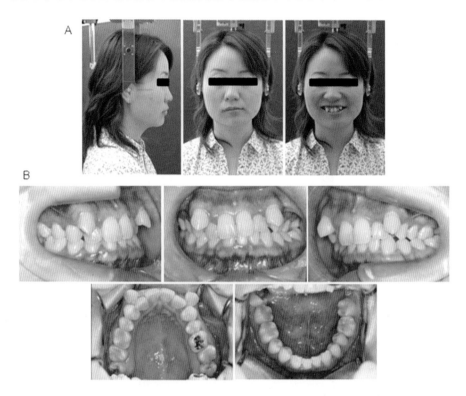

Fig. 15.9 Jaw deviation in a patient with temporomandibular joint dysfunction. (A) Pre and Postoperative photographs of patient with jaw deviation from temporomandibular joint dysfunction. (B) Corresponding photographs of patient's dentition. (From Takigawa Y, Tanikawa C, Yashiro K, et al. Improvement in three-dimensional facial configuration and jaw motion following surgical orthodontic treatment of a case with jaw deviation. *Orthod Waves*. 2017;76(3):184–196 [Fig. 1]. ISSN 1344-0241, https://doi.org/10.1016/j.odw.2017.04.001, http://www.sciencedirect.com/science/article/pii/S1344024117300055)

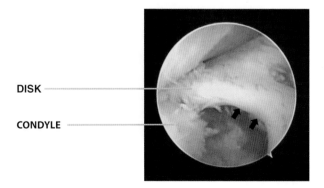

Fig. 15.10 Arthroscopic view of left temporomandibular joint in a patient with severe pain on mastication. Osteoarthritis with disc perforation and exposed condyle. *Black arrow* indicates disc perforation. (From Israel HA. Internal derangement of the temporomandibular joint: new perspectives on an old problem. *Oral Maxillofac Surg Clin North Am*. 2016;28(3):313–333, Fig. 4.)

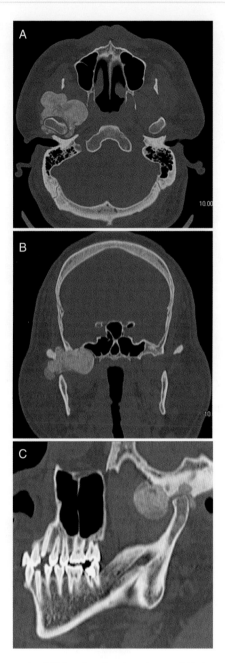

Fig. 15.11   Computed tomography (CT) imaging showing a large calcified mass around the right tempo-romandibular joint (TMJ). (A) Axial CT scan showing a ring-shaped calcified mass around the condylar process of the right TMJ; the mass is not continuous with the mandibular condyle. (B) Coronal CT scan revealing a calcified mass in the joint space; bone resorption and thinning of the middle cranial base are present, and the lesion appears to extend into the middle cranial fossa. (C) Sagittal CT scan of the right TMJ; the calcified mass limits condylar head movement. (From Kudoh K, Kudoh T, Tsuru K, et al. A case of tophaceous pseudogout of the temporomandibular joint extending to the base of the skull. *Int J Oral Maxillofac Surg.* 2017;46(3):355–359, Fig. 1.)

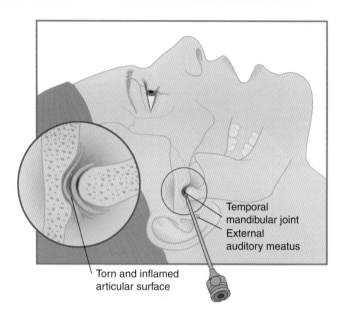

Temporal mandibular joint

External auditory meatus

Torn and inflamed articular surface

Fig. 15.12   Correct needle placement for injections of the temporomandibular joint. (From Waldman SD. *Atlas of Pain Management Injection Techniques.* Philadelphia: Saunders; 2000:5.)

face should also be considered in any patient presenting with ill-defined facial pain after trauma, infection, or central nervous system injury. The pain of TMJ dysfunction is dull and aching, whereas the pain of reflex sympathetic dystrophy of the face is burning, with significant allodynia often present. Stellate ganglion block may help distinguish the two pain syndromes because the pain of reflex sympathetic dystrophy of the face readily responds to this sympathetic nerve block, whereas the pain of TMJ dysfunction does not. In addition, the pain of TMJ dysfunction must be distinguished from the pain of jaw claudication associated with temporal arteritis (see Chapter 11).

TREATMENT

The mainstay of therapy is a combination of drug treatment with tricyclic antidepressants, physical modalities such as oral orthotic devices and physical therapy, and intraarticular injection of the joint with small amounts of local anesthetic and steroid. Antidepressant compounds such as nortriptyline at a single bedtime dose of 25 mg can help alleviate sleep disturbance and treat any underlying myofascial pain syndrome. Clinical experience suggests that selective serotonin reuptake inhibitors, selective serotonin and norepinephrine inhibitors, and atypical selective serotonin reuptake inhibitors may have a role in treating the substrate of anxiety that is often present in patients suffering from TMJ pain.

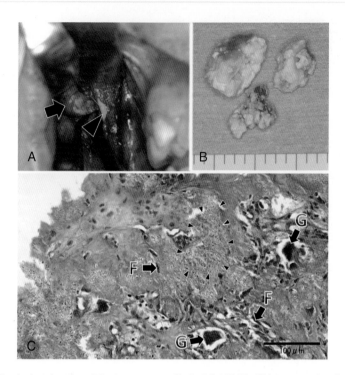

Fig. 15.13 Surgical exploration of the temporomandibular joint (TMJ). (A) Intraoperative view of a mass in the TMJ region showing the deposition of a chalky calcified material *(arrow)*. The *arrowhead* points directly to the right coronoid process of the mandible. (B) The specimen appears white and chalklike. (C) Histologic examination of the specimen showing deposits of crystals *(arrowheads)* in fibrous tissue (stained with hematoxylin-eosin). The crystal deposits consist of rod-shaped and rhomboid crystals, which are surrounded by foreign body—type giant cells *(G)* and fibroblasts *(F)*. (From Kudoh K, Kudoh T, Tsuru K, et al. A case of tophaceous pseudogout of the temporomandibular joint extending to the base of the skull. *Int J Oral Maxillofac Surg.* 2017;46(3):355—359, Fig. 2.)

Orthotic devices help the patient avoid jaw clenching and bruxism, which may exacerbate the clinical syndrome. Intraarticular injection with local anesthetic combined with steroid is useful to palliate acute pain to allow physical therapy as well as to treat joint arthritis that may contribute to the patient's pain and joint dysfunction. The intraarticular injection of platelet-rich plasma may also be beneficial in the treatment of TMJ dysfunction. Clinical studies suggest that the injection of type A botulinum toxin into the temporalis and masseter muscles may also provide symptomatic relief. Rarely, surgical treatment of the displaced intraarticular disc is required to restore the joint to normal function and reduce pain.

For intraarticular injection of the TMJ, the patient is placed in the supine position with the cervical spine in the neutral position. The TMJ is identified by asking the patient to open and close the mouth several times and palpating the area just anterior and slightly inferior to the acoustic auditory meatus. After the joint is identified, the patient is asked to hold the mouth in the neutral position. A total

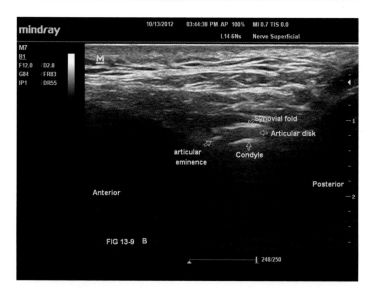

Fig. 15.14   Sonographic anatomy of the temporomandibular joint and surrounding structures.

of 0.5 mL of local anesthetic is drawn up in a 3-mL sterile syringe. When treating TMJ dysfunction, internal derangement of the TMJ, or arthritis or other painful conditions involving the TMJ, a total of 20 mg methylprednisolone is added to the local anesthetic with the first block; 10 mg methylprednisolone is added to the local anesthetic with subsequent blocks. After the skin overlying the TMJ is prepared with antiseptic solution, a 1-inch, 25-gauge styletted needle is inserted just below the zygomatic arch directly in the middle of the joint space. The needle is advanced approximately 0.25 to 0.75 inch in a plane perpendicular to the skull until a pop is felt, indicating that the joint space has been entered (see Fig. 15.12). After careful aspiration, 1 mL of solution is slowly injected. Injection of the joint may be repeated at 5- to 7-day intervals if symptoms persist. Ultrasound needle guidance may improve the accuracy of needle placement and decrease needle-related complications when performing injection of the TMJ (Figs. 15.14 and 15.15).

COMPLICATIONS AND PITFALLS

The vascularity of the region and the proximity to major blood vessels lead to an increased incidence of postblock ecchymosis and hematoma formation, and the patient should be warned of this potential complication. Despite the region's vascularity, intraarticular injection can be performed safely (albeit with an increased risk of hematoma formation) in the presence of anticoagulation by using a 25- or 27-gauge needle, if the clinical situation indicates a favorable risk-to-benefit ratio. These complications can be decreased if manual pressure is

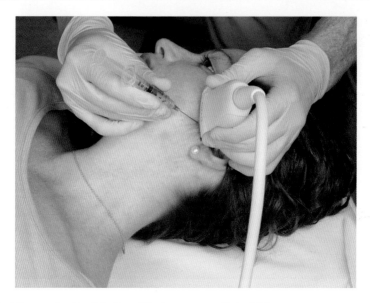

Fig. 15.15 Ultrasound-guided injection of the temporomandibular joint.

applied to the area of the block immediately after injection. Application of cold packs for 20 minutes after the block also decreases the amount of postprocedural pain and bleeding. Another complication that occurs with some frequency is inadvertent block of the facial nerve with associated facial weakness. When this occurs, protection of the cornea with sterile ophthalmic lubricant and patching is mandatory.

HIGH-YIELD TAKEAWAYS

- The patient is afebrile, making an acute infectious etiology unlikely.
- The patient's pain is unilateral and poorly localized to the TMJ.
- The pain has an onset to peak of hours.
- The pain is aching in character.
- The patient has damage to the occlusal surfaces of the teeth due to bruxism.
- Stress can play a part in the evolution of TMJ dysfunction.
- There are no red flags.

Suggested Readings

Dursun O, Çankaya T. Assessment of temporomandibular joint dysfunction in patients with stroke. *J Stroke Cerebrovasc Dis.* 2018;27(8):2141–2146.

Hosgor H. The relationship between temporomandibular joint effusion and pain in patients with internal derangement. *J Cranio-Maxillofac Surg.* 2019;47(6):940–944.

Jenzer AC, Jackson H, Berry-Cabán CS. Temporomandibular joint pain presentation of myocardial ischemia. *J Oral Maxillofac Surg.* 2018;76(11):2317.e1–2317.e2.

Rajapakse S, Ahmed N, Sidebottom AJ. Current thinking about the management of dysfunction of the temporomandibular joint: a review. *Br J Oral Maxillofac Surg.* 2017;55(4):351–356.

Waldman SD. Temporomandibular joint dysfunction. In: *Atlas of Common Pain Syndromes.* 4th ed. Philadelphia: Elsevier; 2019:42–46.

Waldman SD. Temporomandibular joint injection. In: *Atlas of Pain Management Injection Techniques.* 5th ed. Philadelphia: Elsevier; 2021:238–239.

Page numbers followed by "*f*" indicate figures, "*t*" indicate tables, and "*b*" indicate boxes.